DOORWAY THOUGHTS

Cross-Cultural Health Care for Older Adults

**From the Ethnogeriatrics Committee of the
American Geriatrics Society**

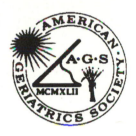

JONES AND BARTLETT PUBLISHERS
Sudbury, Massachusetts
BOSTON   TORONTO   LONDON   SINGAPORE

Jones and Bartlett Publishers

World Headquarters
Jones and Bartlett Publishers
40 Tall Pine Drive
Sudbury, MA 01776
978-443-5000
info@jbpub.com
www.jbpub.com

Jones and Bartlett Publishers Canada
2406 Nikanna Road
Mississauga, ON L5C 2W6
CANADA

Jones and Bartlett Publishers International
Barb House, Barb Mews
London W6 7PA
UK

American Geriatrics Society

Executive Vice President: Linda Hiddemen Barondess
Associate Vice President, Operations, Governance, and
 Communications: Jill Epstein
Manager, Operations, Governance, and
 Communications: Julie Pestana

American Geriatrics Society
The Empire State Building
350 Fifth Avenue, Suite 801
New York, NY 10118
(212) 308-1414
www.americangeriatrics.org

Production Credits
Chief Executive Officer: Clayton Jones
Chief Operating Officer: Donald W. Jones, Jr.
President: Robert W. Holland, Jr.
V.P., Design and Production: Anne Spencer
V.P., Manufacturing and Inventory
 Control: Therese Bräuer
V.P., Sales and Marketing: William Kane
Publisher: Kimberly Brophy
Associate Managing Editor: Carol Brewer

Associate Production Editor: Karen Ferreira
Production Assistant: Carolyn Rogers
Director, Marketing: Alisha Weisman
Director, Interactive Technology: Adam Alboyadjian
Cover and Text Design: Anne Spencer
Composition: Bookwrights
Printing and Binding: Malloy

The procedures and protocols in this book are based on the most current recommendations of responsible medical sources. The American Geriatrics Society and the publisher, however, make no guarantee as to, and assume no responsibility for the correctness, sufficiency, or completeness of such information or recommendations. Other or additional safety measures may be required under particular circumstances.

This textbook is intended as a guide to the appropriate procedures to be employed when rendering medical care to the geriatric population. It is not intended as a statement of the standards of care required in any particular situation, because circumstances and the patient's physical condition can vary widely from one case to another. Nor is it intended that this textbook shall in any way advise medical personnel concerning legal authority to perform activities or procedures discussed. Such local determination should be made only with the aid of legal counsel.

Notice: The patients described in the Case Studies throughout this text are fictitious.

© 2004 by American Geriatrics Society

Library of Congress Cataloging-in-Publication Data
Doorway thoughts : cross-cultural health care for older adults / from the Ethnogeriatrics Steering Committee of the American Geriatrics Society.
  p. ; cm.
 Includes bibliographic references and index.
 ISBN 0-7637-3338-5 (pbk. : alk. paper)
 1. Minority aged--Medical care--Cross-cultural studies. 2. Minority aged--Health and hygiene. 3. Aged--Cross-cultural studies. 4. Gerontology--Cross-cultural studies. 5. Minority aged--Services for.
 [DNLM: 1. Geriatrics--United States. 2. Cross-Cultural Comparison--United States. 3. Health Services for the Aged--United States. 4. Minority Groups--Aged--United States. 5. Professional-Patient Relations--Aged--United States. WT 30 D691 2004] I. Title: Cross-cultural health care for older adults. II. American Geriatrics Society. Ethnogeriatrics Steering Committee.
 RA564.8.D66 2004
 362.6'1'0973--dc22
                    2004004946

Printed in the United States of America
09 08 07 06 05 04   10 9 8 7 6 5 4 3 2 1

CONTENTS

Acknowledgments

The editors wish to thank everyone involved in the development of *Doorway Thoughts*: the authors who gave so generously of their time and experience in writing each chapter; the Ethnogeriatrics Committee of the AGS, whose hard work and dedication paved our way; the AGS Board of Directors, committee chairs, and members for their invaluable comments and suggestions; Jerry C. Johnson, MD, AGSF, for his expert assistance in developing this publication as a whole; David Reuben, MD, AGSF, for his enthusiasm, and promotion of the project; our medical editor Barbara Reitt, PhD, ELS(D); Deviani Maher, MD, FRCPC, for her kind and knowledgeable assistance in developing case studies; and Jill Epstein, Julie Pestana, and the AGS staff, who encouraged and supported every step of this process.

Reva N. Adler
Hosam K. Kamel

Introduction

As the cultural diversity of the elderly age group in the United States continues to grow, it will become increasingly important for clinicians caring for older adults to develop an understanding of different ethnic groups in order to effectively care for their patients in this multicultural society. The purpose of this text is to provide guidelines and assistance to clinicians whose patients include older adults from one or more of these minority groups.

This first chapter discusses the issues and concerns that would apply to clinical encounters with an older person from any minority cultural group. The other chapters address the same issues and concerns, but less generically, providing relevant details regarding the beliefs, traditions, and customs, of seven different groups: African Americans, American Indians and Alaska Natives, Asian Indian Americans, Chinese Americans, Hispanic Americans, Japanese Americans, and Vietnamese Americans. Texts covering other groups will be added in the future. Each chapter is written by a clinician and educator who is either from the same background or who works extensively with a particular ethnic or cultural minority. Each author thus brings to the project a rich combination of scholarship and experience, providing invaluable insight on which readers can draw.

It is very important to keep in mind while using this text that, although the cultural beliefs and characteristics ascribed to each group are accurately described, wide differences appear among the individuals in each group, and each person is unique. Furthermore, the degree of acculturation of older persons from similar backgrounds ranges along a broad spectrum. The culturally astute clinician will remain alert to the differences among individual patients and families from a given culture and on guard against stereotyping an older person on the basis of his or her ethnic or cultural affiliation.

CHAPTER 1

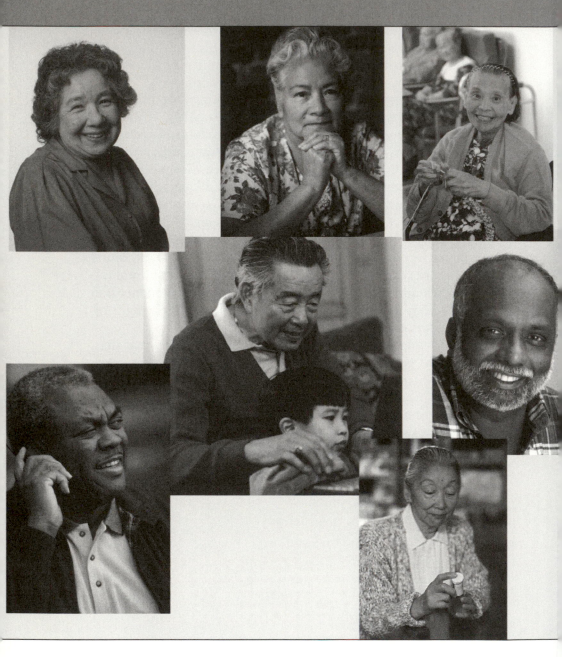

Introduction to Cross-Cultural Health Care for Older Adults

Doorway Thoughts

The key concepts discussed in this text are "doorway thoughts"—factors that the culturally competent practitioner reflects upon before walking through the doorway of any examining, consultation, or hospital room. These factors can shape intercultural health care encounters and relationships for good or for ill. Cultural and historical facts and issues relating to the members of an entire minority group can be in play in any cross-cultural encounter or relationship. The practitioner should be sensitive to the possibility that they may affect their relations with individual patients and families and may also affect patients' willingness or ability to understand, accept, and adhere to prescribed regimens.

The quality of any encounter between a clinician and a patient from different ethnic or cultural backgrounds depends on the clinician's skill and sensitivity. Questions about the individual patient's attitudes and beliefs should be worked naturally and carefully into the clinical interview. Remember that no culture is monolithic. Attitudes and beliefs vary widely from one individual to another within a single cultural group. Prior familiarity with a patient's cultural background will not suffice, for it is inaccurate to assume that a person's outlook is inflexibly linked to his or her cultural heritage. The concepts presented in this text are intended to serve as guides in choosing appropriate questions, rather than a rigid list of cultural attributes or clinical scenarios.

"Doorway thoughts" are factors that the practitioner reflects upon before interacting with a patient.

Preferred Terms for Cultural Identity

The terms referring to specific cultural or ethnic groups can change over time, and individuals in any one group do not always agree on the terminology that is appropriate. It is important to learn what the individual patient's preferred term is for his or her cultural identity and to use that terminology in conversation with the patient, as well as in his or her health records.

Formality
Attitudes regarding the appropriate degree of formality in a health care encounter differ widely between cultural groups. Learning what a new patient's preferences are with regard to formality and allowing that preference to shape the relationship is always advisable. Initially, a more formal approach is likely to be appropriate.

Addressing the Patient
The patient's correct title (e.g., Dr., Reverend, Mr., Mrs., Ms., Miss) and his or her surname should be used unless and until he or she requests a more casual form of address. Another important issue is to determine the correct pronunciation of the person's name.

Addressing the Health Provider
It is also important to learn how the patient would prefer to address the clinician and to allow his or her preference to prevail. For example, in some cultures, trust in the physician depends on his or her assuming an authoritative role, and informality would undermine the patient's trust. This is an aspect of the clinical relationship where the clinician's personal preferences can be relinquished.

Language and Literacy
- What language does this individual feel most comfortable speaking? Will a medical interpreter be needed?
- Does this patient read and write English? Another primary language? If so, which one(s)?
- If the patient is not literate, does he or she have access to someone who can assist at home with written instructions?

It is worthwhile to consider these questions early in the health care relationship to determine whether interpretation services are needed and to make certain that communication with the patient is effective. The clinician should remember that even those who use English fluently may wish to discuss complicated issues in their native language. It is the clinician's responsibility to explain medical terms and to ask the patient for explanations of any cultural or foreign terms that are unfamiliar.

Respectful Nonverbal Communication

Body position and motion is interpreted differently from one cultural group to another. Specific hand gestures, facial expressions, physical contact, and eye contact can hold different meanings for the patient and the clinician when their cultural backgrounds differ. The clinician should watch for particular body language cues that appear to be significant and that might be linked to cultural norms that are important to the patient, in order to cultivate a sensitivity to the conditions that make the flow of communication feel easy and effective.

Early in a relationship with a patient, or when in doubt, the clinician should adopt conservative body language (assume a calm demeanor, avoid expressive extremes such as very vigorous handshakes, a loud and hearty voice, many hand gestures or, on the other hand, an impassive facial expression, avoidance of eye contact, standing at a distance) and remain alert for signals that the person is comfortable or uncomfortable. Directly asking the patient questions about body language may also help. It is very important to avoid making negative judgments about a patient that are rooted in unconscious cultural assumptions about the meaning of his or her gestures, facial expressions, or body language.

The distance from others that individuals find comfortable varies, depending in part on their cultural background. The clinician should determine what distance seems to be the most comfortable for each patient and, whenever practicable, allow the patient's preference to establish the optimal distance during the encounter.

> *Early in a relationship with a patient, or when in doubt, the clinician should adopt conservative body language.*

Elephants in the Room

Are there any issues that are critical to the success of the health care encounter that are present but that go unspoken? The clinician must be alert for the possibility that such issues are indeed present. Examples include:

- A lack of trust in health care providers and the health care system
- A fear of medical research and experimentation
- Fear of medications or their side effects
- Unfamiliarity or discomfort with the Western biomedical belief system

In other chapters, these topics are covered in detail as they relate to specific cultural groups. In general, sensitivity to the possibility that such issues are in play is advised in all intercultural patient encounters.

History of Traumatic Experiences

Is the patient a refugee or survivor of violence or genocide? Are family members missing or dead? Have patients or family members been tortured? Such experiences could negatively affect the health care encounter without the clinician's knowledge unless relevant questions are included among standard questions about the patient's history.

It is important for clinicians to remember that in some historical periods and jurisdictions, health care providers have participated in torture and genocide. For example, in concentration camps during World War II, Nazi medical personnel were responsible for selecting individuals for gassing, supervising the gassing process, and administering lethal injections to inmates in "hospitals." The methods and tools of torture employed have sometimes resembled legitimate clinical procedures and tools. Patients surviving such experiences may not feel safe in medical settings, and contact with all clinicians may invoke feelings of vulnerability, fear, panic, or anger. Great sensitivity is necessary in providing health care for these individuals.

Immigration Status

Some individuals may be residing in North America without the protection of appropriate immigration documents. Clinicians may wish to assure each patient that information given within the medical encounter will be kept in the strictest confidence.

History of Immigration or Migration

The history of the movements of a whole ethnic or cultural group can affect the attitudes and behavior of an individual in that group even when he or she has not immigrated to North America from another country. In addition, understanding the specific migration history of a person often provides insight into the key life transitions informing his or her outlook. Knowing how a person came to reside in North America can be important. The time and effort the clinician invests in learning more about a minority group's history and current situation can be repaid not only in a better relationship with the individual patient but also in an enhanced appreciation of the factors affecting clinical relationships with all patients from that group.

Acculturation

Acculturation is defined as a process in which members of one cultural group adopt the beliefs and behaviors of another group. Acculturation of a group may be evidenced by changes in language preference, adoption of common attitudes and values, and gradual loss of separate ethnic identification. Although acculturation typically occurs when a minority group adopts the habits and language patterns of a dominant group, acculturation may also be reciprocal between groups.

It is essential to keep principles of acculturation in mind during any intercultural health encounter. Begin by determining how long a person has lived in North America and whether he or she was born here. However, remember that the degree to which the person is acculturated to Western customs and attitudes is the consequence of many factors, and not just of the number of years since he or she immigrated. Older adults who follow the traditions of their cultural group may have been born outside of the United States or Canada, may be recent arrivals to the continent, or may even be lifelong North American residents.

A patient's level of acculturation may greatly impact not only his or her health behavior but also preferences in end-of-life planning and decision making. Acculturation can also be an issue dividing family members, and a person's resistance to or ease of acculturation may be a matter of pride or shame and guilt. Developing sensitivity about the issues of acculturation for one's older minority patients is a key element in effective intercultural health care. Asking patients directly about their adherence to cultural traditions can be useful.

Tradition and Health Beliefs

People from non-Western cultural groups may not conceive of illness in Western terms. Some may have highly developed concepts of the causes of health and disease that are incompatible with the concepts that form the foundations of Western medicine. Non-Western paradigms include beliefs that illnesses have spiritual causation or are the result of imbalance among bodily humors, or that they are caused by a person's actions in past lives, to name but a few.

Patients may be making unexamined assumptions that are based on traditional beliefs, and these can cause confusion or create misunderstanding. The more the clinician knows about specific traditions, the more he or she can avoid such problems.

In addition, the clinician should remain alert to the possibility that patients holding such beliefs may be using alternative remedies (e.g., rituals, herbal preparations) that they may not mention, and questions about such practices should be included among other questions about the patient's history. It is unrealistic to expect that a patient will simply "adapt" to Western biomedical approaches to health and health care, just as it is impractical to expect the clinician to accept a new paradigm of wellness and disease. Clinical communication and efficacy will be enhanced when patients and providers make an effort to negotiate a common understanding of causation, diagnosis, and treatment for a specific health problem while maintaining respect for the beliefs and constructs of both individuals.

> *People from non-Western cultural groups may have beliefs about the causes of health and disease that differ from those of Western medicine.*

Use of North American Health Services

Some minority patients may feel uncomfortable in customary North American health care settings. Explanations for the discomfort, distrust, or uneasiness of some include lack of familiarity with Western medical practices, dissatisfying previous encounters with the health care system, or the belief that insensitivity or discrimination is inevitable for anyone in the cultural or ethnic group. Such feelings may result from having been stereotyped or treated insensitively or even unfairly by health professionals in the past. Sensitive exploration of these issues with patients is often both worthwhile and necessary. Individual chapters in this text provide suggestions for possible approaches to patients in specific cultural groups. Generally, the clinician meeting a new patient from an ethnic or cultural minority group should be alert for signs of guardedness that signal an underlying lack of comfort or trust.

Culture-Specific Health Risks

Epidemiologic and medical research has identified numerous differences among ethnic and cultural populations with regard to specific health risks. The clinician who treats many patients from a specific group is advised to make every effort to stay abreast of the latest findings in relevant areas. In the specific chapters of this text, the prevailing thinking about such risks for each group is reviewed.

Approaches to Decision Making

The influence of specific cultures on approaches to health decision making has been the subject of many studies. Western bioethics emphasize individual autonomy in all health decisions, but for many other cultures decision making is family or community centered. Autonomy principles allow competent persons to involve others in their health decisions or to cede those rights to a proxy decision maker. The clinician should ask patients if they prefer to make their own health decisions or if they would prefer to involve or defer to others in the decision-making process. Some may wish to assign the decision-making authority wholly to another individual or a group. In some cultures, the definition of family may include *fictive kin* (people who are considered family despite having no blood relation). In families where the degree of acculturation of the generations differs, the older person may defer to or depend on younger relatives even though the tradition might suggest that the reverse would occur.

Establishing an understanding of each patient's decision-making preferences early in the clinical relationship will, in most instances, promote better communication and avoid the difficulties inherent in trying to address these issues at a time of crisis. When the patient's and clinician's cultural backgrounds differ, careful exploration of these issues is all the more important because the clinician cannot proceed if clinician and patient are not starting from a point of shared understanding.

Disclosure and Consent

Cultural attitudes toward truth telling and disclosure of terminal diagnoses vary widely. In some cultures, it is commonly believed that patients should not be informed of a terminal diagnosis,

In some cultures, it is believed that patients should not be informed of a terminal diagnosis.

as this may be injurious to health or hasten death. Obtaining informed consent in such cases may prove to be difficult. There is no consensus in bioethics concerning the rigorous application of full clinical disclosure in every situation. However, it is generally agreed that incorporating a patient's beliefs concerning disclosure and truth-telling into clinical planning whenever possible is desirable. Some patients may prefer not to know if they are terminally ill and ask that family members or other caregivers receive all diagnostic information and make all treatment decisions. It is advisable to explore each patient's preferences regarding disclosure of serious clinical findings early in the clinical relationship and to reconfirm these wishes at intervals.

Gender Issues

Each culture has intricate traditions and structures with regard to gender roles. Societies seemingly based on the same patriarchal or matriarchal model may vary widely in their expressions of the model. A person's gender will have influenced the sorts of experiences he or she has had, not only within the family but in the community and health care system as well. Another level of complexity may be added to health care encounters when an older adult's group struggles with conflicting traditional and contemporary views on gender roles. Cultural norms for men and women can profoundly influence their health behavior, and these norms for the genders vary widely from one culture to another. These norms also affect decision making, disclosure, and consent.

It is highly advisable for the clinician to explore each patient's attitudes regarding the interplay among gender, autonomy, and personal decision making early in the patient-provider relationship, to confirm his or her preferences at intervals, and to follow the individual patient's wishes whenever possible.

End-of-Life Decision Making and Care Intensity

Culture is an important influence in a person's formation of his or her attitudes toward supportable quality of life, approach to suffering, beliefs about medical feeding, life-prolonging treatments, and palliative care. Some cultures value a direct struggle for life in the face of death, and both patients and families will expect an intensive approach to treatment. Other cultures ardently avoid direct confrontation of death and dying and will prefer to leave such decisions to the clinician. Still others will take a direct approach to death and dying but will reject a too-aggressive approach.

Research has shown that physicians and patients from shared cultural backgrounds have similar values in these areas; the implications of such findings for clinicians and patients from differing backgrounds are obviously important. Both physicians and patients bring their own attitudes and beliefs to any clinical encounter. It is important for clinicians to be aware of their personal views and cultural set when discussing end-of-life plans with patients and to respect patients' beliefs and preferences even when they are different from their own.

In negotiating end-of-life directions with a patient whose background is different from his or her own, the clinician must listen especially carefully to the patient's goals and concerns and exert every effort to avoid making culture-based assumptions that do not apply. For example, the assumption that "no one would want to live in that condition" or that "everyone would want treatment in this situation" is likely to be faulty. To ensure that end-of-life plans and decisions reflect an individual's rights and wishes, the clinician must strive to understand the older person's overall approach to life and death and, as far as possible, provide care that is congruent with that approach.

In the chapters on specific cultural or ethnic groups, the authors provide data from the health services literature regarding the general preferences of a group for end-of-life decisions, life-sustaining care, and advance directives. These data are intended to provide general guidance rather than absolute rules for clinicians when they are discussing end-of-life issues with patients and caregivers from different cultural backgrounds.

Use of Advance Directives

The use of advance directives and health care proxies has become more common in the past 20 years, but research indicates that the use of written directives may be more common among older persons in the dominant North American culture than among older persons in minority cultural groups. It is advisable in intercultural situations, when discussing attitudes and beliefs regarding written directives with a patient, to be sensitive to the possibility that some older persons will prefer to use alternatives—verbal directives or directives dictated to family members or others—and others will need to avoid any such discussion in order to observe proscriptions against talking about death. In view of the fact that preferences for care intensity may also differ according to cultural background, patients should also be given the opportunity to indicate the interventions they do want as well as those they do not want in any written or verbal directive used.

Cultural Competence: A Final Word

There is no gold standard definition of "cultural competence." Most definitions emphasize a careful coordination of individual behavior, organizational policy, and system design to facilitate mutually respectful and effective cross-cultural interactions.

Cultural competence combines attitudes, knowledge base, acquired skills, and behavior. It is an approach, not a technique. Cultural competence is not a form of "political correctness." Ideally, it is a nuanced understanding of the determining role that culture plays in all of our lives and of the impact culture has on every health care encounter, for both the clinician and the patient.

Cultural competence cannot be achieved exclusively by reading, but we hope that this text will provide clinicians who care for older persons from all minority groups with basic information and a foundation for further investigation.

Cultural competence is an approach, not a technique.

We would encourage clinicians to view each intercultural encounter as an opportunity to learn more, not only about the individual patient and his or her culture, but also about themselves. The authors also recommend that clinicians learn more about the impact of culture on health decisions by reading the publications listed in the bibliography, exploring available Web sites, and attending workshops. We also urge clinicians to work with the entire interdisciplinary health care team, including administrators, to promote cultural competence in the health care organizations where they practice. Finally, we encourage clinician educators to develop their own teaching materials and educational programs specifically designed to meet the needs of specific communities.

Reva N. Adler, MD, FRCPC

References

Adelman RD, Greene MG, Charon R, Friedman E. Content of elderly patient-physician interviews in the medical primary care encounter. *Communication Research* 1992;19(3):370–380.

Beisecker AE. Aging and the desire for information and input in medical decisions: patient consumerism in medical encounters. *Gerontologist* 1988;28(3): 330–335.

Beisecker AE, Beisecker TD. Patient information-seeking behaviors when communicating with doctors. *Med Care* 1990;28(1):19–28.

Blackhall LJ, Murphy ST, Frank G, et al. Ethnicity and attitudes toward patient autonomy. *JAMA* 1995;274(10):820–825.

Braun KL, Nichols R. Cultural issues in death and dying. *Hawaii Med J* 1996; 55(12):260–264.

Braun KL, Nichols R. Death and dying in four Asian American cultures: a descriptive study. *Death Stud* 1997;21(4):327–359.

Burke G. Ethics and medical decision-making. *Prim Care* 1980;7(4):615–624.

Caralis P, Davis B, Wright K, et al. The influence of ethnicity and race on attitudes toward advance directives, life-prolonging treatments, and euthanasia. *J Clin Ethics* 1993;4(2):155–165.

Charles C, Gould M, Chambers L, et al. How was your hospital stay? patients' reports about their care in Canadian hospitals. *CMAJ* 1994;150(11): 1813–1822.

Clark JA, Potter DA, McKinlay JB. Bringing social structure back into clinical decision making. *Soc Sci Med* 1991;32(8):853–866.

Cotton P. Talk to people about dying—they can handle it, say geriatricians and patients. *JAMA* 1993;269(3):321–322.

Eleazer GP, Hornung C, Egbert C, et al. The relationship between ethnicity and advance directives in a frail older population. *J Am Geriatr Soc* 1996;44(8): 938–943.

Emanuel EJ, Emanuel LL. Four models of the physician-patient relationship. *JAMA* 1992;267(16):2221–2226.

Finucane TE, Shumway JM, Powers RL, et al. Planning with elderly outpatients for contingencies of severe illness: a survey and clinical trial. *J Gen Intern Med* 1988;3(4):322–325.

Fox SA, Stein JA. The effect of physician-patient communication on mammography utilization by different ethnic groups. *Med Care* 1991;29(11):1065–1082.

Garrett JM, Harris RP, Norburn JK, et al. Life-sustaining treatments during terminal illness: who wants what? *J Gen Intern Med* 1993;8(7):361–368.

Goold SD, Arnold RM, Siminoff LA. Discussions about limiting treatment in a geriatric clinic. *J Am Geriatr Soc* 1993;41(3):277–281.

Green, JW. *Cultural Awareness in the Human Services: A Multi-Ethnic Approach*. Boston: Allyn and Bacon; 1998.

Hall JA, Roter DL, Katz NR. Meta-analysis of correlates of provider behavior in medical encounters. *Med Care* 1988;26(7):657–675.

Hare J, Nelson C. Will outpatients complete living wills? a comparison of two interventions. *J Gen Intern Med* 1991;6(1):41–46.

Harwood A, ed. *Ethnicity and Medical Care*. Cambridge, MA: Harvard University Press; 1981.

Haug MR. Doctor-patient relationships and the older patient. *J Gerontol* 1979; 34(6):852–860.

Haug MR, Ory MG. Issues in elder patient-provider interactions. *Res Aging* 1987;9(1):39–44.

Helman CG. *Culture, Health and Illness: An Introduction for Health Professionals*. 3rd ed. Oxford, UK: Butterworth-Heinemann Ltd; 1994.

High D. Advance directives and the elderly: a study of intervention strategies to increase use. *Gerontologist* 1993;33(3):342–349.

Hypertension Detection and Follow-up Program Cooperative Group. Five-year findings of the Hypertension Detection and Follow-up Program: II: mortality by race-sex and age. *JAMA* 1979;242(23):2572–2577.

Janofsky JS, Rovner BW. Prevalence of advance directives and guardianship in nursing home patients. *J Geriatr Psychiatry Neurol* 1993;6(4):214–216.

Jennings, B. Cultural diversity meets end-of-life decision making. *Hosp Health Netw* 1994;68(18):72.

Jensen J. Trust in doctor deters elderly from seeing other providers. *Mod Healthc* 1986;16(9):49–50.

Kalish RA, Reynolds DK. *Death and Ethnicity: A Psychocultural Study*. Los Angeles, CA: University of Southern California Press; 1976.

Kim SS. Ethnic elders and American health care—a physician's perspective. *West J Med* 1983;139(6):885–891.

Klessig J. The effect of values and culture on life-support decisions. *West J Med* 1992;157(3):316–322.

Levy DR. White doctors and black patients: influence of race on the doctor-patient relationship. *Pediatrics* 1985;75(4):639–643.

Lipson, JG, Dibble SL, Minarik PA, eds. *Culture and Nursing Care: A Pocket Guide*. San Francisco, CA: UCSF Nursing Press; 1996.

Marcus AC, Reeder LG, Jordan LA, et al. Monitoring health status, access to health care, and compliance behavior in a large urban community: a report from the Los Angeles health survey. *Med Care* 1980;18(3):253–265.

Murphy S, Palmer J, Azen S, et al. Ethnicity and advance care directives. *J Law Med Ethics* 1996;24(2):108–117.

Palafox N, Warren A, eds. *Cross-Cultural Caring: A Handbook for Health Care Professionals in Hawaii*. Honolulu, HI: Transcultural Health Care Forum; 1980.

Reilly BM, Magnussen CR, Ross J, et al. Can we talk? inpatient discussions about advance directives in a community hospital: attending physicians' attitudes, their inpatients' wishes, and reported experience. *Arch Intern Med* 1994;154 (20):2299–2308.

Roter DL, Hall JA, Katz NR. Patient-physician communication: descriptive summary of the literature. *Patient Education and Counseling* 1988;12:99–119.

Rubin SM, Strull WM, Fialkow MF, et al. Increasing the completion of the durable power of attorney for health care: a randomized, controlled trial. *JAMA* 1994;271(3):209–212.

Sachs GA, Stocking CB, Miles SH. Empowerment of the older patient? a randomized, controlled trial to increase discussion and use of advance directives. *J Am Geriatr Soc* 1992;40(3):269–273.

Satcher D. Does race interfere with the doctor-patient relationship? *JAMA* 1973;223(13):1498–1499.

Schmerling RH, Bedell SE, Lilienfeld A, et al. Discussing cardiopulmonary resuscitation: a study of elderly outpatients. *J Gen Intern Med* 1988;3(4):317–321.

Schonwetter RS, Teasdale TA, Taffet G, et al. Educating the elderly: cardiopulmonary resuscitation decisions before and after intervention. *J Am Geriatr Soc* 1991;39(4):372–377.

Silverman H, Tuma P, Schaeffer M, et al. Implementation of the patient self-determination act in a hospital setting: an initial evaluation. *Arch Intern Med* 1995;155(3):502–510.

Smucker WD, Ditto PH, Moore KA, et al. Elderly outpatients respond favorably to a physician-initiated advance directive discussion. *J Am Board Fam Pract* 1993;6(5):473–482.

Szasz TS, Hollender MH. The basic models of the doctor-patient relationship. *Arch Intern Med* 1956;97:585–592.

Teno J, Fleishman J, Brock DW, et al. The use of formal prior directives among patients with HIV-related diseases. *J Gen Intern Med* 1990;5(6):490–494.

Terry M, Zweig S. Prevalence of advance directives and do-not-resuscitate orders in community nursing facilities. *Arch Fam Med* 1994;3(2):141–145.

Uhlmann RF, Pearlman RA, Cain KC. Understanding of elderly patients' resuscitation preferences by physicians and nurses. *West J Med* 1989;150(6):705–707.

Vaughn G, Kiyasu E, McCormick WC. Advance directive preferences among subpopulations of Asian nursing home residents in the Pacific Northwest. *J Am Geriatr Soc* 2000:48(5):554–557.

Veatch RM. Models for ethical medicine in a revolutionary age: what physician-patient roles foster the most ethical relationship? *Hastings Cent Rep* 1975; 2(3):3–5.

Vukmir RB, Kremen R, Dehart DA, et al. Compliance with emergency department patient referral. *Am J Emerg Med* 1992;10(5):413–417.

Waitzkin H. Doctor-patient communication: clinical implications of social scientific research. *JAMA* 1984;252(17):2441–2446.

Ware JE Jr, Bayliss MS, Rogers WH, et al. Differences in 4-year health outcomes for elderly and poor, chronically ill patients treated in HMO and fee-for-service systems: results from the Medical Outcomes Study. *JAMA* 1996;276(13):1039–1047.

Yeo G, Hikoyeda N, McBride M, et al. *Cohort Analysis as a Tool in Ethnogeriatrics: Historical Profiles of Elders from Eight Ethnic Populations in the United States.* Stanford GEC Working Paper #12. Stanford, CA: Stanford Geriatric Education Center; 1998.

CHAPTER 2

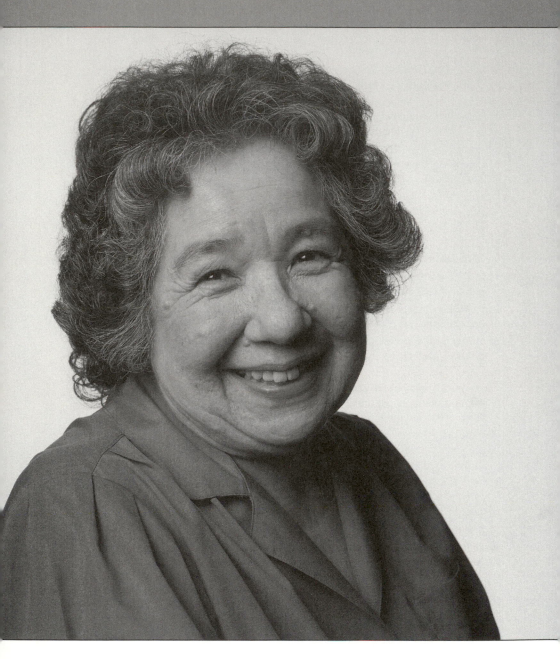

Older American Indians and Alaska Natives

Doorway Thoughts

The clinician should communicate an attitude of honor for the American Indian or Alaska Native elderly person. (Hereafter, for the sake of brevity, both groups are referred to as American Indians or Indians.) It is considered an honor to be involved in the life of an older person from this community in any way. Communicate this by thanking the patient for the opportunity to try to help him or her to remain healthy and by attending very closely to the person's words. Allow the older person to speak without interruption, then go back and ask specific questions. Listen closely for topics in the conversation that suggest questions that you might ask in order to learn more about the context of the patient's daily life, whether in a certain tribe or in an urban area away from homelands.

Allow the older person to speak without interruption, then go back and ask specific questions.

Preferred Cultural Terms

For most elderly persons from these groups, the terms *Indian*, *American Indian*, or *Alaska Native* would likely be appropriate. The term *Native American* sometimes connotes a political position that is associated with younger generations. For many individuals, tribal identification coexists with, and often supersedes, identification as Indian.

Formality of Address

A formal mode of address at first is advised. Use titles (e.g., Dr., Reverend, Mr., Mrs., Ms., Miss) unless given permission by the older person to use his or her first name. The elderly Indian person is most likely to address the physician as "Doctor."

Informality is commonly valued, but this attitude may not emerge until a comfortable relationship with the clinician has developed. Also, it is common for older Indian men and women to have great appreciation for humor during social encounters. For some, subtle satirical humor is very highly valued. The injection of humor into the conversation can help establish a social connection with the older Indian person and his or her family.

Language and Literacy

Although most elderly Indian men and women speak English well, others speak it only as a distant second language. Also, many elderly Indians read English, but some live the legacy of limited education in the Western tradition. It would be well to assume that even those who are fluent in English may still want to discuss complicated issues in their native language.

Respectful Nonverbal Communication

During all encounters with elderly Indians, clinicians need to position themselves in a way that shows the elderly person that they are not there to dominate. As with informality in forms of address, informality in personal touching may not be appropriate until a comfortable relationship with the clinician has developed.

History of Traumatic Experiences

There is a general concern in the Indian community that the medical establishment has used American Indians experimentally without informed consent. The clinician should be alert for signs that such fears are affecting the clinical encounter with individual elderly Indians.

During all encounters with elderly Indians, clinicians need to position themselves in a way that shows they are not there to dominate.

Immigration Status

Despite their unique position in the United States as natives of the North American continent, Indians have experienced relocation programs that have left their demographic mark, including concentrations of tribal groups in large urban areas. In addition, frequent movement between home reservations or homelands and urban centers is common. These shifts in location are commonly economically driven and can adversely impact the individual patient's patterns of use of the health care system.

Degree of Acculturation

The cultural identities of American Indians and Alaska Natives vary widely, ranging along a continuum from the traditional to mainstream American culture. Many Indian elderly persons live parts of their lives in very traditional ways, yet these may be concealed from health care providers. There is often no association between "full blood" status and adherence to traditional culture. Likewise, an elderly Indian may be only "part Indian" genetically but observe many traditional values. In addition, the heterogeneity of tribal cultures and among individuals within a specific tribe is great.

Tradition and Health Beliefs

Elderly Indians often integrate traditional concepts such as interaction with nature, balance, and harmony with biomedical health models. The general dynamics of health and disease are believed by Indians to involve the need to maintain or regain a sense of coherence with self, nature, and others, such as family (which is highly variably defined), friends, and community. The restoration of balance is achieved by such means as rituals, personal intent, and herbal remedies. The intent on the part of the healer to do good is also considered to be an important component of the healing process.

For many American Indians, disease is attributed to varying aspects of the nonphysical environment. This may take the form of disease-object intrusion beliefs; that is, the belief that illness results from the insertion of an object into the body by an enemy. The cure is removal by a traditional healer. Or it may take the form of the belief that sickness can be caused by a noncorporeal spirit entity that enters the body and possesses it. Again, the cure is removal by a traditional healer. Another common belief is that the person's spirit or essence has been lost. Traditional healers find and bring the spirit back to the body.

It may be difficult for clinicians to ascertain the extent of an individual Indian patient's use of alternative or traditional medicine. Complicating the matter is the fact that the older Indian man or woman may conceal traditional beliefs in the conviction that traditional medicine and practices are not valued by biomedical health practitioners. Elements of traditional practices may be considered secret or private, and detailed questioning about practices by a biomedical health practitioner may be seen as intrusive.

Use of North American Health Services

The historical experience of American Indians and Alaska Natives with government health programs has profoundly affected the attitudes of many elderly individuals in these groups. The Indian Health Service (IHS) is the primary provider of care for most rural Indian communities. Over half of that care is provided by tribally run health programs, and the IHS itself has become, in recent years, an Indian-operated health system. Nevertheless, at times it is seen as user unfriendly and overburdened. High professional staff turnover often inhibits the development of personal relationships between patients and clinicians and may exacerbate an underlying fear that Indian people are receiving suboptimal care. Conversely, Indian patients may be quite loyal to what they perceive as "their" hospital or clinic.

The individual Indian patient's adherence to traditional health beliefs may well be accompanied by a deep skepticism toward biomedical practices and an all-too-great familiarity with the limitations of the health care system.

Culture-Specific Health Risks

Type 2 diabetes mellitus is of epidemic proportion in Indian country, with attendant end-organ injury resulting in increased rates of coronary artery disease, blindness, renal failure, and limb amputation. Dementia, reported by many to be rare among Indian people, is certainly present. Elders with dementia are often not identified by family as "ill" or "lost," but, rather, changed in capability and function. They often retain an important role in family life.

Approaches to Decision Making

Many decisions are made in a family unit that includes people outside the immediate nuclear family. The family boundaries may be extensive and favor some specific kinsmen, such as a mother's brother or paternal aunts. Often, however, with widespread urban relocation and the presence of fewer people on reservations, traditional patterns of family organization among Indians have been altered. Decision-making for many elderly Indian men and women may be difficult when the person(s) authorized under traditional structures to make decisions for the elder live elsewhere.

Disclosure and Consent

Honesty on the part of the clinician is highly valued, as is carefulness about obtaining consent for treatment. These issues are best understood in the context of the historical experience of a population that has experienced genocidal policies at times and that still encounters suboptimal treatment in some health care settings.

At the same time, the requirement to be honest does not suggest the need to be aggressively direct in the delivery of bad news. Honest directness may be prized. One can talk about "a growth" rather than "cancer" and convey that biomedical practice has reached the limits of its ability to cure without making a statement about incurability. The need to convey prognosis honestly should be met while still conveying hopefulness. Predictions of life expectancy in the absence of imminent death may be regarded as ill intentioned or, in some way, contributing to death.

The need to convey prognosis honestly should be met while still conveying hopefulness.

Gender Issues

Attitudes about gender roles are highly varied, depending on the individual patient's tribal culture, kinship patterns, and social experience. For example, most tribes are known to define family membership either by the mother's or the father's line. Consequently, for example, an older person's mother's relatives may be differentially involved in health decision making if the mother's family line is used as the family membership reference point for the patient. However, this does not mean that for tribes that use the mother as the reference point, women have the dominant social power. Similarly, for tribes that use the father's family line to define family membership, the males do not necessarily possess the dominant social power.

There may also be socially accepted gender roles that supersede tribal and contemporary social conventions. For example, the social role of a "strong woman" is one that recognizes a person's exceptional social power and influence. Such a woman may be important for sanctioning health activities in a given community.

It is also expected in many tribes that people will significantly identify with the gender role changes found in contemporary American society. Traditional gender-specific role behavior may be muted in younger adults but more persistent among the elderly adults in the same community.

End-of-Life Decision Making and Care Intensity

The clinician who provides health care for American Indian and Alaska Native elderly persons should remember a number of key points relating to decisions about end-of-life care and care intensity:

- Any limitation of care may be seen as an attempt to unfairly ration care.
- Tribal cultures that value the struggle for life in the face of death may show ardent avoidance of the discussion of death and dying.
- Decision making may require the presence of certain family members; in their absence, the family member or members who are present may not feel authorized to make decisions.
- Decision-making capacity may not rest solely with the older person, but may be a process involving other family members.
- There is generally no expectation that interventions that will not help the older person should be done.
- The benefits of staying on homeland and with family may outweigh the desire to "have everything done" if this requires transferring an elderly relative to a tertiary care center; this may be particularly true for the oldest-old.

Use of Advance Directives

Advance directives have posed problems for clinicians and institutions providing care for American Indian elders because this approach may not be consistent with the culturally prescribed ways of talking about death. Even in the face of death and preparations for death, families may maintain a positive, hopeful outlook. A fruitful approach strives to understand the elderly person's overall approach to life and death and seeks to provide care that is consistent with that. Family members can be of great help in defining an appropriate approach. There are no shortcuts. The clinician should avoid any approach that demands that older adults or families "confront" or discuss death or a terminal diagnosis in a prescribed manner.

| CASE STUDY **1** | **Getting to Know You** |

Objectives

1. Examine your personal communication style and approach based on your culture's values, beliefs, and behaviors.
2. Discover how your personal communication style will change when working with individuals from different cultures.
3. Discuss approaches to balancing the ethical principle of personal autonomy (stressed in Western medical ethics) with the principle of family responsibility and cohesion (present in many other cultural ethical systems).
4. Realizing that no culture is homogeneous, discuss your approach to understanding the impact of culture on each of your individual patients.

Michael Miller, MD, is a family medicine physician, who is practicing in an Indian health service clinic on an American Indian nation. Dr. Miller comes from Connecticut, owes 2 years of clinical service to the Indian Health Service, and has been on duty for 5 days. Today, Dr. Miller is seeing Maggie Smith, a 70-year-old American Indian female patient, for a follow-up visit regarding her diabetes. Mrs. Smith comes in today with two of her six grandchildren and one of her four daughters. Mrs. Smith is married, lives on the reservation, and speaks only her traditional language. Mrs. Smith has no formal Western education, but is renowned within her tribe for her healing practices and her cultural wisdom.

Questions:

1. What questions might you have as a physician interacting with an individual from a culture with which you are not familiar?
2. What questions might you have as a patient when interacting with a physician that is not of your culture?

Dr. Miller enters the room and introduces himself to the patient in English. The patient is seated in a chair next to the desk that Dr. Miller takes. After his brief introduction, he immediately begins by asking Mrs. Smith what brings her into the clinic today. Mrs. Smith gives him a puzzled look and does not respond.

Questions:

1. What communication issues arise in this brief scenario?
2. How would you improve on Dr. Miller's approach?

Mrs. Smith's daughter informs Dr. Miller that Mrs. Smith speaks only her traditional language. Dr. Miller then requests that the daughter serve as the interpreter for the clinical interaction and also requests that the grandchildren not be present because of his concern of confidentiality.

Questions:

1. What are the limitations of family or friend interpreters? What are the specific limitations from an American Indian point of view, if any?
2. When non-English-speaking patients come to your practice, how do you and your organization address this? If on-site interpretation services are not available to you and your patients, what strategies might you use?
3. What two types of information, other than translation of "words," occur during professional medical interpretation?

An interpreter is identified who is not a family member. The interpreter informs Dr. Miller that the patient would like the grandchildren to remain in the room with her daughter. With the interpreter present, the clinical interaction moves along with greater ease.

Two weeks later, Joey, one of Mrs. Smith's grandchildren, is brought in by his mother. Dr. Miller shakes the mother's hand, greets the child and his mother in English, and asks what brings them to the clinic. They immediately proceed to give Dr. Miller a detailed history of Joey's recent illness, including fever, pain in the right ear, and vomiting. Dr. Miller prescribes rest, fluids, acetaminophen, and an antibiotic. The encounter goes very well.

A year passes and Mrs. Smith returns for one of her regular visits with Dr. Miller. He greets her in the traditional style of her tribe and then asks the interpreter to step into the room for the rest of the interview. Mrs. Smith and Dr. Miller have formed a strong working relationship. Her glucose levels are under much better control and she is feeling quite well.

Question:

1. What are some similarities and differences between Dr. Miller's approach to Mrs. Smith and his approach to her children and grandchildren? Include issues of cultural heterogeneity and acculturation in your answer.

| CASE STUDY **2** | **Talking About Dying Without Talking About Death** |

Objectives

1. Examine your expectations about how information relating to death and dying is communicated.
2. Analyze how you would adjust your own communication style to meet the needs of the patient and family.
3. Analyze how your own cultural influences impact your encounters about death and dying with your clients.

Mr. Wood, an 87-year-old American Indian with late stage prostate cancer, is transferred back to his community hospital for palliative care. Since diagnosis, he has received all of his care at a tertiary care center and has not been seen by his community physician or at his home community hospital. There is a cursory transfer note from his oncologist simply stating that there is no further life-prolonging therapy available to Mr. Wood and that he prefers to go home. On evaluation, the admitting physician finds a thin, frail, ill-appearing elder, surrounded by family. He converses with family members in his native language, but speaks with the physician in English. The eldest son is identified as the family spokesperson.

Question:

1. How would you initiate a conversation with Mr. Wood concerning his health and his wishes for future care?

Outside of the room, the admitting physician asks the son whether his father knows that he has cancer, that the cancer has progressed, and that the plan for this admission is to focus on comfort measures. The son responds initially that his father does not know that he has cancer and is not "expecting to die." Anxiously, the physician asks, "Should we talk with him about this so that he can make the plans he needs to make and we can be sure he gets the care he needs?" The son responds calmly, "He is already making plans. He's telling us who should get the house, who should get the tractor, how he should be buried."

Questions:

1. Autonomy is the principle in Western medical ethics that dictates that individuals should make their own health decisions. How is Mr. Wood demonstrating his autonomy? What type of communication plan could meets his needs?
2. What cultural influences do you draw on when you think about the "correct" ways to discuss death and dying? How does your thinking affect your practice? How would your influences impact your approach to Mr. Wood in an intercultural discussion about death and dying?

The physician understands that although the elder and his family are not talking about the imminence of his death and are not doing anything that might hurry it along, they are well aware of it and are making appropriate arrangements. A care plan is established to focus on palliation and is explained to the patient and his family, without ever explicitly discussing the imminence of his death. He dies peacefully, with family present, 2 months later.

Bruce S. Finke, MD
J. Neil Henderson, PhD (Oklahoma Choctaw)
Melvina McCabe, MD (Navaho)

References

Avery C. Native American medicine: traditional healing. *JAMA* 1991;265(17): 2271–2273.

Burhansstipanov L. Urban Native American health issues. *Cancer* 2000;88(5 Suppl):1207–1213.

Green JW. *Cultural Awareness in the Human Service: A Multi-Ethnic Approach.* Boston: Allyn and Bacon; 1998.

Henderson JN, Henderson LC. Cultural construction of disease: a "supernormal" construct of dementia in an American Indian tribe. *J Cross-Cultural Gerontol* 2002;17:1–16.

Jennings B. Cultural diversity meets end-of-life decision making. *Hosp Health Netw* 1994;68(18):72.

McCabe M. Health care of American Indian/Alaska Native elders. In: Galloway JM, Goldberg BW, Alpert JS, eds. *Primary Care of Native American Patients.* Boston: Butterworth-Heinemann; 1999;323–332.

Rousseau P. Native-American elders: health care status. *Clin Geriatr Med* 1995; 11(1):83–95.

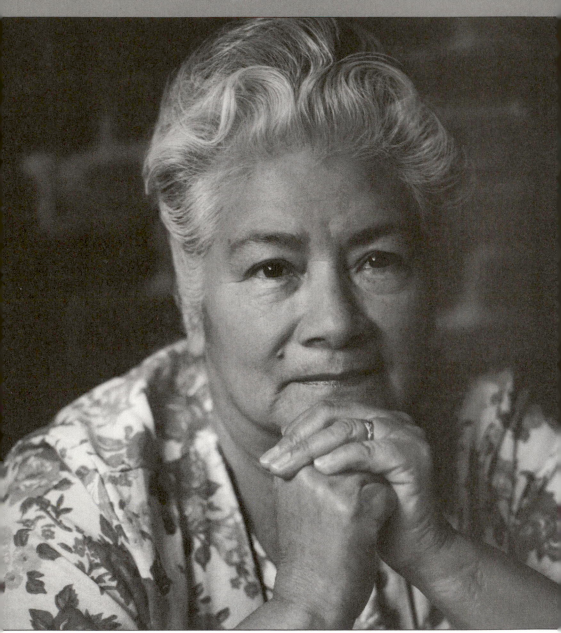

CHAPTER 3

Older Hispanic Americans

Doorway Thoughts

Elderly Hispanic Americans in the United States are a diverse group. The majority is of Mexican origin, but new immigrant populations from other parts of the Caribbean and Central and South America are accounting for an increasing proportion of this growing population.

Preferred Cultural Terms

Some older Hispanic Americans may not use the term *Hispanic*; instead, terms that designate the country of origin may be more readily embraced. Other terms frequently used include *Latino, Latino American, Mexican American, Cubano, Puerto Riqueño,* or *Chicano*. For the sake of brevity, this text uses *Hispanic* and *Hispanic American* to designate all the groups. The clinician caring for Hispanic American elders is advised to ask each patient about his or her preference with regard to cultural designation.

Formality of Address

One of the important values in Hispanic tradition centers on the treatment of individuals with trust, respect, and dignity; Hispanics expect to be treated with respect and dignity regardless of job or social status. Hispanic American elders therefore tend to be more formal during their initial interaction with a clinician and expect to be addressed by their title (e.g., Mr. or Mrs., or Sr. or Sra.). They often hold health care professionals in high regard, and they usually value the professional opinions of their clinicians.

Treat patients with respect and dignity regardless of job or social status.

To enhance communication and decision making with Hispanic elders, clinicians need to begin the relationship in a formal, polite manner and, once rapport is established, to express a genuine "kinship" with the patient. Touching and hugging may ultimately be acceptable, as is asking about family or loved ones. The relationship between older Hispanics and clinicians is best when it is based on *personalismo* (the inclination to relate and trust individuals as opposed to systems or organizations). Thus, the bond is typically between the older Hispanic patient and the individual clinician, and not the clinic or institution.

Language and Literacy

Fifty percent of older Hispanic Americans report that they speak English well. Among Hispanic Americans, older Cubans who immigrated just prior to the Castro era are the most educationally privileged. The newly immigrated older Mexicans tend to have had fewer years of formal education. It may be helpful to provide Spanish-language educational materials in a variety of presentations, including textual as well as illustrated-story formats.

Respectful Nonverbal Communication

Hispanic women may not like a firm handshake, even though they will shake hands upon introduction. They also may not be accustomed to maintaining continuous eye contact, especially with male clinicians. It may be advisable to lower eyes frequently during interviews with older Hispanic women.

Patterns of Immigration

Hispanic Americans make up the second largest group of ethnic elderly persons in the United States, comprising an estimated 5% of the population aged 65 years and older. This group is diverse, originating from different nationalities, cultures, and classes. Hispanics immigrated to the United States from Mexico, Cuba, Puerto Rico, and Central and South America. An Hispanic individual may be descended from a variety of ethnic groups, including Africans, Native Americans, and Spanish colonizers. Given these additional ethnic modifiers, the term *Hispanic* is far from definitive, glossing over important variations. It only very generally describes a person who has a Spanish surname, is Spanish-speaking, or has a birthplace in a Spanish-speaking country.

Degree of Acculturation

Acculturation has been defined as an adaptive process of cultural adjustments whereby individuals change their life condition. As with other immigrant populations, acculturation among Hispanic elders tends to be reflected in changes in their language and social interactions. Age plays an important role in the degree of acculturation. Persons who immigrated at an older age often have more difficulty making cultural adjustments than do those who immigrated at a younger age.

The best approach is to ask each patient about his or her experience. Initial questions might include "Where were you born?" and "How long have you lived in this country?" If the clinician is unsure how acculturated the patient is, it is all right to admit ignorance by saying, "I have noticed that some (Mexican, Cuban, Puerto Rican, Guatemalan, . . .) patients are very traditional whereas others are more Americanized. Which group do you believe you belong to?"

Tradition and Health Beliefs

Traditional Hispanics believe that the world is inhabited by both good and evil spirits that may affect the person in a positive or a negative way. The Mexican system of *curanderismo*, the Cuban system of *santería*, and the Puerto Rican system of *espiritismo* all have beliefs related to these special powers at work in the world. These belief systems are also sources of alternative medicine. The use of these modalities tends to wane as individual Hispanics become more integrated in the Eurocentric model that is dominant in the United States. One study of elderly Mexican Americans found their use of folk remedies to be far lower than that reported by other groups.

Culture-Specific Health Risks

Statistically, patients of Hispanic origin, like those from other minority groups, are less likely to be referred for screening procedures, such as mammography, or to receive advanced surgical procedures. The culturally sensitive clinician will be alert to such disparities and discuss appropriate screening tests with older Hispanic patients. Hispanic patients also tend to receive less information than their white counterparts and are more likely to receive a lower quality of care.

Hispanic patient tend to receive le information than their white counterparts and are more likely to receive a lower quality of care.

Among Mexican American elders, acculturation has been associated with a decline in the prevalence of many diseases, including hypertension and diabetes mellitus. It has also been linked to their increased ability to cope with outside stressors and to their decreased morbidity.

Elephants in the Room

Hispanic elders feel more comfortable with clinicians of a similar cultural background for reasons of language, cultural connection, and shared knowledge of traditional health practices, but development of trusting intercultural patient-provider relationships is certainly possible. The growth of trust depends in part on the clinician's sensitivity to several social factors. Even as the number of elderly Hispanic Americans continues to grow, their access to health care services remains limited; some experts have suggested that English proficiency may be an important factor limiting access. Socioeconomic disadvantages have also been proposed as reasons for limited access. In addition, some Hispanic Americans lack American job skills and may feel powerless after years of poverty and perceived discrimination. It is also important to remember that Hispanic American immigrants to the United States have lived through periods when they were segregated by culture, race, and socioeconomic status.

Approaches to Decision Making

Family relations are greatly valued in the Hispanic culture. Most Hispanics are socialized in the belief that the needs of the family are more important than the needs of the individual. This value places the emphasis on cooperation and sharing and thus leads to the family's being the most important support system for older Hispanics. However, as each generation becomes acculturated to the American value system and fewer people live in extended family households, the cultural expectations of older Hispanics for family support often go unmet.

Besides emphasizing mutual social responsibility, the Hispanic family structure also tends to be patriarchal. The oldest male tends to be the decision maker as well as the authority figure. Additionally, religious life often plays a central role in Hispanic family culture and may affect health decision making. Although many Hispanics no longer are Roman Catholic, theirs remains a predominantly Christian culture. Clinicians may wish to include attention to the relationship between prayer and healing in their discussion with Hispanic families of critical health decisions.

Hispanics generally focus on the present rather than the future. This value helps the social unit focus on problems at hand. This time orientation differs from the Eurocentric view that emphasizes future time and problems yet to come. The Hispanic elder's tendency to value concentration on the present may present some difficulty in medical decision making, especially with regard to those decisions concerning potential future outcomes.

Six elements have been proposed as essential for good health-related decision making: mutual respect for the interests and needs of both doctor and patient; ability of the patient and physician to access each other for consultation; adequate understandable information for each on the health issues involved; mutual willingness to make and accept necessary referrals; reassurance about the appropriateness of each individual's behavior; and a specific, mutually agreed-upon course of action. For older Hispanic patients, the assumption that all these elements are present may not be valid. Carp reminds clinicians that "the old, poor, and members of ethnic minority groups have relatively little in common with the mainstream of society and are in poor communication with it."

Disclosure and Consent

Hispanic elders come to their physicians expecting them to do what is appropriate for them. They also expect to be treated with justice. It is important for physicians to understand the cultural value of *personalismo* before attempting to deliver bad news. Hispanic patients place a great value on getting to know their physicians. Spending time with the older Hispanic patient to allow a level of trust to develop and to break through the formality of the doctor-patient relationship is necessary before delivering bad news. It is also important to spend time with the patient and his or her family after delivering bad news to show the "personal touch." Elder Hispanics and their families place great value on this component of the doctor-patient relationship.

It is important to spend time with the patient and his or her family after delivering bad news.

Gender Issues

Many Hispanics observe traditions of *machismo* and *marianismo*, which provide the gender roles for males and females, respectively. *Machismo* refers to a patriarchal system of male authority and leadership which specifies that men should be strong, in control, and live by a code of honor. In the United States, many elderly Hispanic men experience frustration because of their inability to live according to this ideal. *Marianismo* refers to the ideal woman as being like the Virgin Mary, who is restrained, submissive, self-sacrificing, and spiritual. While outwardly dependent and docile, Hispanic females are the managers of the home and in the United States may be considered more valuable in the job market.

End-of-Life Decision Making and Care Intensity

When a clinician discusses end-of-life issues with a patient, any ethnic, religious, and cultural differences between them can become crucial. Sound end-of-life decisions depend on a good relationship and open communication between the clinician and the patient and family. Hispanic American elders rely more heavily on family and physician input than do their white counterparts when it comes to end-of-life decisions.

A palliative approach to care at the end of life may be acceptable, but disapproval of assisted suicide is strong among Mexican American elders; in one study, close to two-thirds of Mexican Americans surveyed disapproved of legalizing assisted suicide, and more than 70% felt that assisted suicide was wrong. Bedolla says that Mexican American elders are guided primarily by the ethical principles of beneficence, nonmaleficence, and justice and not by the principle of autonomy. This suggests that individuals may choose to yield some of their personal autonomy when issues of beneficence and nonmaleficence are involved.

Religious faith may be a significant factor influencing end-of-life decision making among Hispanics. Hispanic elders are predominantly Roman Catholic, and their views may reflect the Roman Catholic Church's strong stand against assisted suicide and increasing acceptance of palliative care. However, Mouton et al. did not find religious faith to be linked to Mexican Americans' strong opposition to assisted suicide in the context of a terminal illness; this opposition may reflect a cultural rather than religious construct.

Use of Advance Directives

As with end-of-life discussions, Hispanic American elders rely more heavily on the family's and physician's input than do non-Hispanic whites, which may make it difficult to elicit a completely autonomous decision from the patient. Relatives of the older Hispanic man or woman commonly demand an aggressive treatment approach, apparently for fear of abandonment. There is evidence to indicate that even when elderly minority patients prefer a palliative approach to care, they rarely communicate this to their physicians. Feelings of trust and comfort with the physician are likely to enhance doctor-patient communication on end-of-life issues.

Ethnicity is also strongly associated with knowledge of and attitudes toward advance directives. Caralis et al. showed in a study of middle-aged adults (mean age 51 years) that more Hispanics (42%) than whites (14%) want their doctors to keep them alive regardless of how ill they are. Mexican Americans are also less likely than whites to believe that patients should make decisions about the use of life support.

Mexican Americans tend to make decisions in the context of the family, with several family members participating in end-of-life discussions. Although these family members may participate, the final decision rests with a single family member.

One explanation for any lack of communication between the Hispanic elder and his or her clinician may be the historically limited access to health care for ethnic minority groups. Hispanic patients may be afraid of not receiving care at all if they limit life-sustaining therapies. Those with difficulty accessing the health care system may interpret discussions about withholding life-sustaining therapy as further barriers to obtaining care. Another explanation may be that clinicians often do not incorporate religious beliefs about end-of-life issues into their discussions, nor do they typically solicit pastoral input into end-of-life decision making.

Mexican Americans tend to make decisions in the context of the family, with several family members participating in end-of-life discussions.

The culturally sensitive clinician will be alert to these issues and may wish to assure patients that do-not-resuscitate orders will in no way abridge access to all other treatment modalities. It is also advisable to establish mutual agreements with patients regarding the use of advance directives and end-of-life decision making as the clinical relationship progresses, well in advance of emergency situations. Reassurance that care will continue to be provided often facilitates the communication of a desire for a palliative approach.

| CASE STUDY **1** | **The Interplay of Faith and Healing** |

Objectives
1. Describe how the spiritual beliefs of an older Hispanic patient may impact both his or her health behavior and the health care encounter.
2. Understand your own inner spiritual beliefs and describe how they may affect your interactions with patients whose beliefs differ from yours.

Dr. DeLeon is a middle-aged, Mexican American geriatrician practicing in a long-term care setting affiliated with an urban teaching hospital. She was raised and educated in the United States, and her Spanish language capabilities are limited. She is a practicing Episcopalian.

Alicia Rosales is a 69-year-old Roman Catholic woman, originally from El Salvador, who is now living in the same city. She speaks English at a grade-school level. Mrs. Rosales, her husband, and another couple are involved in a weather-related, multiple-car accident. Mrs. Rosales awakens from surgery to find that in addition to the loss of her spouse and the other couple, she has lost her left leg. Her extended family lives in another state. During her hospital stay, she remains quiet, speaking little to her physicians, the nursing staff, social workers, or pastoral care team. She is discharged to a skilled nursing facility (SNF) for ongoing wound care for her left above-knee amputation, and physical rehabilitation.

Dr. DeLeon visits her for the first time for a full admission history and physical examination after Mrs. Rosales has been transferred to the SNF. She learns about Mrs. Rosales' accident and losses from the hospital discharge summary. She enters the room with some trepidation, not sure how to broach the subject of the deaths of her patient's companions. Instead, she introduces herself in English and asks whether or not Mrs. Rosales' pain is well managed. She receives a brief reply that yes, it is. The rest of the interview is similarly terse. During the physical exam, Mrs. Rosales follows directions, but is noncommunicative. Dr. DeLeon is sure that Mrs. Rosales is experiencing pain, both physical and psychological, but is unsure how to break through her patient's stoicism.

Questions:
1. How would you approach Mrs. Rosales' reticence to discuss her pain and feelings of grief and loss?
2. How does the principle of *personalismo* relate to the relationship between Dr. DeLeon and Mrs. Rosales?

Just before leaving the room, Dr. DeLeon speaks for the first time in Spanish. She has not spoken in Spanish previously, because she is self-conscious about what she considers her mediocre vocabulary and marginal grasp of verb conjugation. She is, however, desperate to offer the new widow a gentle condolence about the loss of her husband and friends.

Questions:
1. How might the use of Spanish language skills, even if limited, improve a health care encounter with an older Hispanic patient? What cultural principle does this reflect?
2. How does the loss of Mrs. Rosales' spouse and the lack of extended family in the area affect her health decision making?

"Pues, se me hace que Usted tiene un santo para cuidarle," meaning to infer that Mrs. Rosales' husband is now in heaven to watch over her. Mrs. Rosales' face lights up. She reaches into her pocket and pulls out a medallion with the image of a saint on it. *"Sí! Él me protegió!"* (Yes! He protected me!) Startled by this sudden and animated response to the statement about saints in general that she mistakenly made, Dr. DeLeon responds, *"Quizas Dios tiene algún trabajo para Usted,"* (suggesting that perhaps God had more work for Mrs. Rosales to do, and therefore spared her). This mention of God causes Mrs. DeLeon to dissolve in tears. She launches into a stream of conversation about her grief, her family, her pain, and also her faith. Dr. DeLeon and Mrs. Rosales eventually design a treatment plan for the pain, and the doctor promises Mrs. Rosales that a priest will visit to give her communion. Nursing staff later report that Mrs. Rosales is requesting pain medication when needed and is communicating well in English concerning her needs.

Questions:
1. What value system(s) did Dr. DeLeon use to gain Mrs. Rosales' confidence? How do faith and religious belief interact with medical practice for many Hispanic Americans?
2. How would you interact with a patient, such as Mrs. Rosales, who has strong religious convictions?

Mrs. Rosales is soon transferred to an SNF in the state where her relatives live. Prior to discharge, she tells Dr. DeLeon that she will get better quickly so that she can embark upon whatever work God has kept her on Earth to do. They hug and say goodbye. Following Mrs. Rosales' arrival in the out-of-state SNF, she progresses rapidly and is discharged to her family's care to complete rehab as an outpatient.

CASE STUDY **2** | **Permiso and Respeto**

> *Objectives*
> 1. Understand the concepts of "respect" and "permission" as they apply to working with older Hispanic patients.
> 2. Be able to obtain pertinent information concerning the cultural beliefs of older Hispanic patients so that an effective treatment plan can be developed.

Dr. Hovander is a 41-year-old English-speaking internist who is bilingual in Spanish because of his studies abroad and the diligent maintenance of his language skills. He practices in an upper-class urban setting which recently has experienced an influx of immigrants from Mexico. He is very comfortable with his language skills and eagerly anticipates speaking Spanish more frequently with his patients. His colleague, Dr. Angela Reyes, is a 38-year-old geriatrician from northern New Mexico who speaks no Spanish aside from a few phrases that she picked up from her parents.

Mr. Trujillo and his wife are descended from early Spanish colonists who settled the Southwest in the fifteenth century. They are fully bilingual in Spanish and English. They recently moved in with their grandson's family, where they cook and help with their great-grandchildren's after-school care. Mr. Trujillo develops headache and anorexia and goes to see Dr. Hovander.

Dr. Hovander is happy to have a client with a Spanish surname and assumes that Mr. Trujillo is from Mexico. His initial interview with Mr. Trujillo is quite focused. The doctor asks questions in Spanish, but Mr. Trujillo answers in English. The doctor then tells him to change into a gown for the examination and leaves the room. When he returns, he begins to examine Mr. Trujillo without any preliminary comments. Mr. Trujillo is increasingly tense. After the examination, Dr. Hovander hands him a prescription and tells him to make a return appointment in 2 weeks, then leaves the room.

Questions:
1. What assumptions does Dr. Hovander make about Mr. Trujillo's country of origin, and how do they affect his communication with his patient?
2. How might Dr. Hovander's behavior be interpreted by Mr. Trujillo with regard to the concept of *respeto* (mutual respect)?

Mr. Trujillo makes a return appointment, but asks to see a different provider. The scheduling desk gives him an appointment with Dr. Reyes.

She reads in his chart that Dr. Hovander has prescribed an antidepressant to treat Mr. Trujillo's symptoms. When she enters the room, Mr. Trujillo immediately starts complaining about the medication he was prescribed: it was too expensive; it tasted bad; it didn't make him feel any better. "I'm not depressed! They don't even know what's wrong with me, so I'm not going to take any of that medicine any more!" he loudly informs the doctor. His affect is angry and belligerent. Dr. Reyes listens to the outburst patiently and then extends her hand to Mr. Trujillo. He takes her hand automatically, but instead of pulling away, Dr. Reyes kneels down beside him and tells him that she is there to listen to him, and that she will value whatever he can tell her about his health because he knows his body better than anyone else ever will. He responds with a derisive snort. Dr. Reyes then asks if he will allow her to examine him. He acknowledges her request with a brief nod.

Questions:

1. What would be an effective approach for Dr. Reyes to obtain further medical history from Mr. Trujillo?
2. What would be an effective approach to the examination of Mr. Trujillo in his present state of dissatisfaction?

Instead of having Mr. Trujillo change into a gown, Dr. Reyes asks him to sit on the examining table in his clothes. She politely asks permission to unbutton the top of his shirt so that she can listen to his heart. She discovers a large religious medallion hanging just above his heart and respectfully asks that he hold it during her examination. She continues the examination using a minimal amount of disrobing and always asks permission before touching any part of Mr. Trujillo's body, warning him that the stethoscope may be cold, explaining where her hands will push, and so on. At the conclusion of the examination, she asks Mr. Trujillo's opinion as to the cause of his symptoms.

"Well, I think I'm worn out from running after those little kids all day long. I'm too tired to think, too tired to eat. I am too old for this! But I don't want to tell my grandson—they have been so good to me and my wife—I don't want to let him down." Dr. Reyes admits that taking care of small children would wear anyone down. She agrees with Mr. Trujillo's refusal of antidepressant therapy. She asks the clinic social worker to join them, and Mr. Trujillo begins to help develop a plan to treat his exhaustion that includes improving the child care arrangements at home.

Questions:

1. How did asking permission enable Dr. Reyes to evaluate her patient? What cultural principle does this reflect?
2. How did Dr. Reyes bridge the previously established communication gap? How did Dr. Hovander's approach differ?

Dr. Hovander notices that Dr. Reyes saw Mr. Trujillo in follow-up and asks her about the outcome of their visit. She describes Mr. Trujillo's reaction to the antidepressant therapy. She also tells of her approach to Mr. Trujillo, which seemed to encourage him to trust and be more involved with planning his care. Dr. Hovander realizes that he still has more to learn about the rich cultural interplay between physicians and Hispanic American elders, which is far more than just learning the language.

Charles P. Mouton, MD, MS

Marie Luz Villa, MD

References

Adams PL. Black patients and white doctors. *Urban Health*. 1977;6(6):21–23.

Bedolla MA. The principles of medical ethics and their application to Mexican-American elderly patients. *Clin Geriatr Med* 1995;11(1):131–137.

Caralis PV, Davis B, Wright K, et al. The influence of ethnicity and race on attitudes toward advance directives, life-prolonging treatments, and euthanasia. *J Clin Ethics* 1993;4(2):155–165.

Carp FM. Communicating with elderly Mexican Americans. *Gerontologist* 1970;10(2):126–134.

Fox SA, Stein JA. The effect of physician-patient communication on mammography utilization by different ethnic groups. *Med Care* 1991;29(11):1065–1082.

Hypertension Detection and Follow-up Program Cooperative Group. Five-year findings of the Hypertension Detection and Follow-up Program: II: mortality by race-sex and age. *JAMA* 1979;242:2572–2577.

Mouton CP, Johnson MS, Cole DR. Ethical considerations with African American elders. *Clin Geriatr Med*. 1995;11(1):113–129.

Teno J, Fleishman J, Brock DW, et al. The use of formal prior directives among patients with HIV-related diseases. *J Gen Intern Med*. 1990;5(6):490–494.

CHAPTER 4

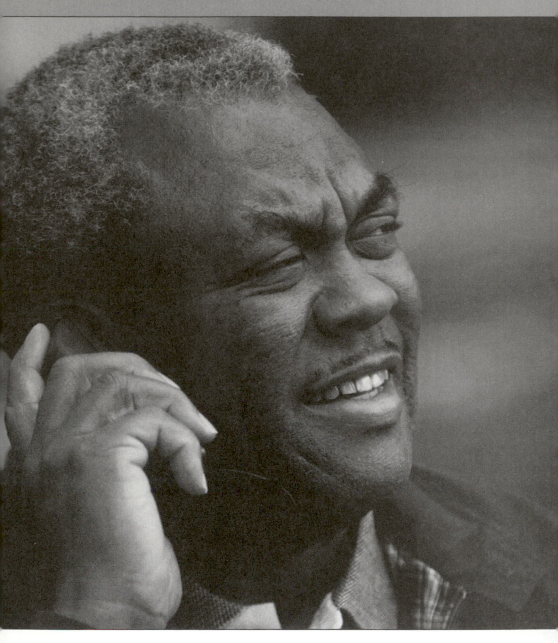

Older African Americans

Doorway Thoughts

The African American or black population in the United States is diverse, with a large degree of intragroup variation. The focus of discussion herein is African American elders who are native to the United States. For comments on others, see the section below on immigration status.

General concepts about African American elders that are described here must be personalized to the individual patient. It is important that generalizations not become stereotypes that are used in defining individual patients.

Preferred Cultural Terms

The current cohort of older African Americans may have been called *colored*, *Negro*, or *black* at various stages of their lives. Individual elders may not have embraced the terms in current use: *African American* or *black*. The terms *colored* or *Negro* are generally offensive to both patients and family members.

Formality of Address

Many African American elders may consider it inappropriate to be addressed by their first name, especially if the clinician is younger and has not been invited to be more familiar. It is advisable, therefore, to address patients by title and surname (e.g., Mr. Jones, Mrs. Johnson, Reverend Smith). Asking the patient or family member how he or she prefers to be addressed is acceptable.

Address patients by title and surname (e.g., Mr. Jones, Mrs. Johnson, Reverend Smith).

Language and Literacy

The literacy levels and language skills of African American elders vary widely, from illiterate to learned, depending on the individual's educational background. Language appropriate to the patient's educational level should always be used. Medical jargon should be avoided and issues should be explained in clear terms, using everyday language. It may be useful to confirm comprehension by asking patients and family members to express, in their own words, their understanding of the discussion. Similarly, the clinician should ask for explanations of words or expressions the patient uses that may be unfamiliar.

Respectful Nonverbal Communication

Nonverbal communication skills are very important. Discussions should be held in a comfortable setting without distractions. Body language from the clinician that encourages dialogue includes sitting close to the bed next to the patient, rather than at the foot of the bed or standing across the room or in the doorway. The clinician should maintain eye contact whenever possible.

Use of North American Health Services

In general, older African Americans seek health care less frequently and at later stages of illness than their white counterparts do. They are also more likely to receive care in settings that do not foster the development of a caring, ongoing relationship with one primary clinician. This means that a trusting, mutually respectful clinician-patient relationship, which needs to be carefully developed and nurtured over time, may not have been a reality for most older African Americans.

Clinicians should be aware that their agenda and that of the patient or family might be very different. It may be very welcoming to ask the patient and family what their expectations are for each health care encounter.

Many older African Americans who receive care in a teaching hospital environment are concerned or fearful that they will be "experimented on" or will receive care from unsupervised trainees. All medical students, residents, and other trainees should be introduced to the patient and family, and their role as members of the health care team should be explained. The attending physician should reassure the patient and family that he or she is involved with all aspects of care.

Immigration Status

The term *African American* is a racial description for black persons living in the United States, a group that includes not only those who were born in the United States but also those with origins in European, Caribbean, African, or South American countries. This discussion focuses on the needs, traditions, and experience of older African Americans native to the United States, including both those with rural backgrounds and those from urban areas. Individuals born outside of the United States are likely to have distinct cultural traditions and attitudes. In these instances, it is advisable to become familiar with the relevant cultural information in order to establish a better clinical relationship.

Tradition and Health Beliefs

The current cohort of African American elders may believe that illness is the result of an imbalance or impurity in their system, perhaps the result of exposure to a draft or eating the "wrong" type of food. Others may feel that their illness is divine retribution for a sin or misdeed; in this instance, an illness may become a testing of faith that requires divine intervention. Still others have health beliefs that are similar to those of their white counterparts in that they are based on the biomedical view of health and disease.

A variety of folk or home remedies may be tried, particularly if the elder has had a life history of limited access to the health care system and few economic resources. Many elders are reluctant to discuss their use of these remedies with their physician, and a significant amount of trust and sensitivity is needed to get a complete history of all treatments the patient may be using.

A significant amount of trust and sensitivity is needed to get a complete history of all treatments the patient may be using.

Culture-Specific Health Risks

Older African Americans are at high risk for a number of chronic illnesses, including hypertension, cardiovascular and cerebrovascular diseases, diabetes mellitus, and osteoarthritis. These diseases may have begun in young adulthood and are now associated with significant end organ damage and disability. Obesity is especially prevalent among older African American women and is an important risk factor for diabetes, cardiovascular disease, and some cancers.

African Americans have high age-adjusted rates for cancers of the prostate, lung, cervix, and esophagus. They also appear to be at an increased risk for Alzheimer's disease and multi-infarct dementia.

Approaches to Decision Making

Family members generally expect to be involved in discussions and decision making. The roles and relationships of all family members should be discussed and clarified. Many older African Americans have fictive kin. These are people who are considered family as the result of longstanding relationships, even though they are not linked by blood ties. In some cases, these persons may play a larger role than true family members in providing care and support for the older person, which may pose a challenge if no formal health care proxy has been designated.

Patients should be asked whom they would choose to make their health care decisions.

Disclosure and Consent

Given the fear of many older African Americans of being used for experiments or being cared for by trainees, it is important that the clinician individualize all aspects of care. Some African American families may request that certain diagnoses or prognoses be withheld from the patient to shelter him or her from disturbing information. Other patients and families favor forthright discussion of all medical issues and treatment plans. The clinician may find that some patients prefer that the family act as the conduit for information, and that direct communication with the patient is limited by the patient's desire not to know the full consequences of the illness. In some instances, the patient may seek information in parcels, and the clinician must allow for ongoing discussion over several visits. It is strongly advised that the clinician discuss these preferences with each patient, but well in advance of urgent health care needs.

The clinician should not assume that an African American elder who asks few questions has no desire for information and is unwilling to give consent. It may be helpful to ask the patient or family about their understanding of the illness and treatment options and to use this as the basis for further discussion.

Gender Issues

Older African American women have generally worked outside of the home for the majority of their lives and have traditionally been responsible for providing economic support for their families, either alongside their husbands or as single heads of the household. Many women are the family matriarchs and may have provided care to children, grandchildren, and other extended family members. They are generally held in high esteem by their families; they are respected for their wisdom and ability to survive despite challenging life circumstances. For married women, health care decisions are generally made in conjunction with spouses.

End-of-Life Decision Making and Care Intensity

Several studies suggest that African Americans are more likely than white Americans to continue aggressive therapies, even when outcomes are expected to be poor. They are also less likely to complete do-not-resuscitate orders or living wills. One explanation for this behavior is a fear that refusing aggressive care may lead to their receiving compromised care.

Patients may fear that refusing aggressive care could lead to their receiving compromised care.

The wishes of patients and family should always be respected. Counseling by either a member of the clergy or a church leader may be helpful. Issues related to end-of-life care should ideally be discussed in the office setting, before the onset of a health crisis and within the bounds of a mutually trusting physician-patient relationship.

Use of Advance Directives

Many African Americans do not feel comfortable about signing a legal document that reduces or changes the care they receive. Religious beliefs may also play a role, in that many older African Americans believe that God is ultimately in control and is the only one who can determine outcomes.

| CASE STUDY **1** | **There's No Place Like Home** |

Objectives

1. Identify standards of courtesy and respect for African American elders.
2. Discuss the key issues in considering DNR status for older African Americans.
3. Be aware of challenges when diagnosing and treating pain within intercultural provider-patient encounters.

Dr. George Houston is a geriatrician in an academic medical center. He is an Italian American who has been a member of the faculty for 5 years. Several times a year, he serves as the attending physician on the inpatient team and is often asked to provide geriatrics expertise to patients on the surgical service.

He is called by one of the attending urologists to do a consult on Lemuel Johnson, an 86-year-old African American male with metastatic prostate cancer. The urology service has been attempting to send the patient to a nursing home with no further hospitalizations, because there are no other interventions to offer the patient at this time. Dr. Houston is called to assist with discharge planning. Mr. Johnson was informed by the urology resident, during morning rounds, that there were no other treatment options for him. Mr. Johnson was upset because the resident repeatedly referred to him as "Lemuel" and talked in a loud voice as though he were hard of hearing. When Mrs. Johnson arrived at the hospital later that morning, the urology team was in the operating room and not available to meet with her to answer her questions. The urology team left a message with the nurse that Mrs. Johnson should select a nursing home for her husband because he was ready for discharge. The Johnsons have also been asked to complete do not resuscitate (DNR) papers as soon as possible.

Mrs. Johnson is fearful that if they sign the DNR papers, the doctors will no longer provide any care to her husband. She is upset that the urologist told her husband that he should not be admitted to the hospital again because nothing else could be done for his cancer. She feels that he is in a great deal of pain, and that the doctors have not been giving him enough pain medication. In addition, Mrs. Johnson does not want her husband in a nursing home. The closest facility is miles from her home and is not located on a convenient bus route. Mrs. Johnson does not drive and cannot afford the taxi fares that would be needed for her to visit her husband. Furthermore, this particular nursing home is run by Jewish Family Services and only offers kosher meals to the residents.

Mr. Johnson requires total care in all activities of daily living, and his needs far exceed that which his elderly wife can provide. She insists, however, that he come home so that she can care for him. Furthermore, Mrs. Johnson refuses to sign DNR papers and wants Mr. Johnson be resuscitated and intubated in the event of a cardiopulmonary arrest.

Mr. Johnson is a retired porter for a now-defunct train company that ran from Florida to New York City. He left school at age 12 to begin working to help support his family. He met his wife during his years on the railroad, and they eventually settled in New York City. Mr. and Mrs. Johnson have been married for 54 years, but they never had children of their own. They did, however, raise Mr. Johnson's two nephews after his sister died. Both children are very devoted to the Johnsons, but have fulltime jobs and families and do not live nearby. They are not able to assist Mrs. Johnson in providing daily care to her husband. Mr. and Mrs. Johnson have been active members of their church for many years. Mrs. Johnson is one of the elder members of the deacon board, and Mr. Johnson was a head usher in the church until his illness.

Dr. Houston enters Mr. Johnson's room and finds Mrs. Johnson at his bedside. He introduces himself and explains that he has been called to help develop a safe discharge plan. Before beginning, he asks Mr. Johnson if he feels up to having a quick physical examination and asks him how he would like to be addressed. Mr. Johnson states that he prefers to be called "Mister Johnson." Dr. Houston examines Mr. Johnson and finds him to be weak, but alert, and in moderate pain. He seems to have normal hearing and is able to respond appropriately to questions. He is thin and has lost more than 30 pounds in the last 2 months. He is bed bound and incontinent, and can eat small amounts, if fed. Dr. Houston's examination indicates a likely prognosis of 6 months or less. He makes a recommendation for liquid morphine with food and fluids as tolerated. Dr. Houston explains to the Johnsons that he will be calling a social worker to assist him in working out a discharge plan. He leaves the room consider how he can best assist this gentleman and his family with Mr. Johnson's end-of-life planning.

Questions:
1. From a cultural perspective, what may the Johnson family have found discourteous in the behavior of the urologist?
2. What cultural issues may have initially made Mrs. Johnson reluctant to sign the DNR papers?
3. How do you think Mrs. Johnson would have described her feelings about her husband's initial pain management?
4. Why might Mrs. Johnson have been reticent to accept hospice care when it was first mentioned?

Dr. Houston is able to contact the geriatric team social worker who arranges a meeting for the next day with Mrs. Johnson, her two children, and the pastor of their church. At first, Mrs. Johnson is reluctant to consider palliative services. Ultimately, they are able to work out a plan by which Mr. Johnson can be discharged home with hospice services. Mrs. Johnson is reassured that, should the need arise, readmission to the hospital for comfort measures is possible under hospice. She feels much better, however, when she learns that hospice can provide most of the care for her husband in their own home. She also likes the fact that physicians and nurses will be available to them at any time and is pleased with his current pain management. She completes the DNR papers and is comforted by the fact that he will be able to die at home. During the meeting, she and her children are able to have all of their questions addressed. The pastor offers additional support for Mrs. Johnson that will be provided by several members of the church. Mr. Johnson is discharged home the next day.

Dr. Houston receives word a week later that Mr. Johnson died peacefully at home surrounded by family and friends.

CASE STUDY **2**	**A Royal Pain in the Neck**

> ### Objectives
> 1. Identify several ways to ensure good intercultural provider-patient communication.
> 2. Examine the barriers to good intercultural medical care in a busy clinical setting.
> 3. Discuss the origins of the distrust that some older African Americans may have with North American health services.

Dr. Meeta Mookerjee is a third-year resident in internal medicine with a busy outpatient practice in an academic medical clinic. She is a first generation Asian Indian who enjoys the outpatient clinic, but feels rushed to complete her sessions quickly so that she can get back to the hospital to work up the new admissions that occur steadily throughout the day.

Essie Mae Bookman is a 79-year-old African American woman who has been a patient of Dr. Mookerjee's for approximately 3 years. She often has to wait an hour or more to be seen and frequently skips appointments if she can't get a ride to the clinic. Her past medical history is significant for hypertension, osteoarthritis of the knees and lower back, obesity, and depression. She comes in today complaining of a cough she has had for about 6 months. The cough is intermittent, but is worse at night when she is in bed. The cough is nonproductive and is not associated with any systemic symptoms. She denies any chest pain or shortness of breath.

Mrs. Bookman retired from the housekeeping department of the local community hospital. She never married, but has one adult daughter and two grandchildren who sometimes bring her to appointments and assist her with shopping and housecleaning tasks. Although she walks with a cane, Mrs. Bookman lives alone and can manage basic activities of daily living independently. She lives in her own home in a declining neighborhood and is very proud of her garden. During the summer, she frequently brings tomatoes and collard greens from her garden to Dr. Mookerjee and the clinic staff.

Mrs. Bookman and her daughter moved to the area from Georgia in the 1940s. She completed sixth grade in the segregated school system of rural Georgia. In her younger days, Mrs. Bookman was known to smoke and drink heavily and used to frequent area bars after work and on weekends. However, she has not smoked or had a drink in more than 25 years. Mrs. Bookman used to attend church regularly, but stopped going several years ago when it became difficult for her to find rides to and from services.

Dr. Mookerjee examines Mrs. Bookman and notes clear lung fields with no wheezes, rales, or rhonchi. There is no adenopathy or evidence of any acute pathology. Dr. Mookerjee orders a chest x-ray, which reveals a large substernal mass. A subsequent MRI of the neck shows a large, multinodular goiter with partial compression of the trachea.

Mrs. Bookman returns for a follow-up appointment to discuss these results and brings her daughter into the room with her. Dr. Mookerjee tells Mrs. Bookman and her daughter of the large, multinodular goiter discovered in her chest and suggests that the next step is a consultation with a surgeon to have the goiter removed. She tells Mrs. Bookman that her risk factors for surgery are low and that she should be able to return to her current level of function and quality of life after the surgery. Dr. Mookerjee goes on to explain that the cough is an indication that the goiter is compressing the trachea and, with time, could cause complete obstruction with severe respiratory distress and death. Dr. Mookerjee's beeper goes off and she leaves the room to answer the call, but sends the nurse in to show Mrs. Bookman and her daughter out.

Mrs. Bookman is scheduled for a surgical evaluation, as well as another follow-up appointment with Dr. Mookerjee for medical clearance prior to surgery. One month later, however, Dr. Mookerjee learns that Mrs. Bookman did not keep her appointment with the surgeon. When she returns with her daughter, Mrs. Bookman readily admits that she did not see the surgeon. She says that because she has cancer, she plans to die "with all the body parts the Lord gave me," and she will not be a subject so that "some young surgical resident can experiment on me" while she is under anesthesia. She states that she does not want anyone cutting her and will not have surgery.

It quickly becomes evident to Dr. Mookerjee that she has not clearly conveyed the situation to Mrs. Bookman and her daughter, both of whom mistakenly believe that Mrs. Bookman has cancer.

Dr. Mookerjee is about to begin clarifying the situation when her beeper goes off. As she is leaving the room, Mrs. Bookman is restating that she is "not some guinea pig for a surgical resident."

Questions:

1. What are some of the factors that contributed to Mrs. Bookman's misunderstanding of her illness?
2. What historical and other factors have led to Mrs. Bookman's fear of medical experimentation in what she initially perceives to be her "situation?"
3. From a cultural perspective, what environmental and interpersonal changes could be implemented in the medical clinic to improve provider-patient communication and care?

This time, Dr. Mookerjee makes a quick call to ask another resident to cover her for a few minutes. She returns to Mrs. Bookman and her daughter and clearly and slowly explains the particulars of a goiter, tracheal compression, and the low risk of cancer. She gives Mrs. Bookman details of the operation, but tells her that the surgeon can answer more specific questions about the actual operation. She is careful to select words and terms that are easy to understand. She frequently stops and asks Mrs. Bookman and her daughter to repeat what they have heard so that she is better able to determine their level of understanding. After 20 minutes, Dr. Mookerjee is satisfied that Mrs. Bookman understands the basic information about her illness.

Mrs. Bookman's daughter encourages her mother to make another appointment with the surgeon and promises to accompany her to the visit. Mrs. Bookman agrees, but states that she is still not interested in having surgery. Dr. Mookerjee calls the surgical clinic and speaks to one of the surgical residents prior to Mrs. Bookman's appointment, to help facilitate the visit.

Sharon A. Brangman, MD, FACP, AGSF

References

Brangman SA. African American elders: implications for health care providers. *Clin Geriatr Med* 1995:11(1) 15–23.

Caralis PJ, Davis B, Wright K, et al. The influence of ethnicity and race on attitudes toward advance directives, life-prolonging treatments, and euthanasia. *J Clin Ethics* 1993;4(2):155–165.

Eleazer GP, Hornung C, Egbert C, et al. The relationship between ethnicity and advance directives in a frail older population. *J Am Geriatr Soc* 1996;44(8): 938–943.

High DM. Advance directives and the elderly: a study of intervention strategies to increase use. *Gerontologist* 1993;33(3):342–349.

Klessig J. The effects of values and culture on life support decisions. *West J Med* 1992;157(3):316–322.

McKinley ED, Garrett JM, Evans AY, et al. Differences in end-of-life decision making among black and white ambulatory cancer patients. *J Gen Intern Med* 1996;11(11):651–656.

Mouton CP, Johnson MS, Cole DR. Ethical considerations with African American elders. *Clin Geriatr Med* 1995:11(1):113–129.

Murphy ST, Palmer JM, Azen S, et al. Ethnicity and advance care directives. *J Law Med Ethics* 1996;24(2):108–117.

Silverman HJ, Tuma P, Schaeffer MM, et al. Implementation of the patient self-determination act in a hospital setting: an initial evaluation. *Arch Intern Med* 1995;155(5):502–510.

Sugarman J, Weinberger M, Samsa G. Factors associated with veterans' decisions about living wills. *Arch Intern Med* 1992;152(2):343.

CHAPTER 5

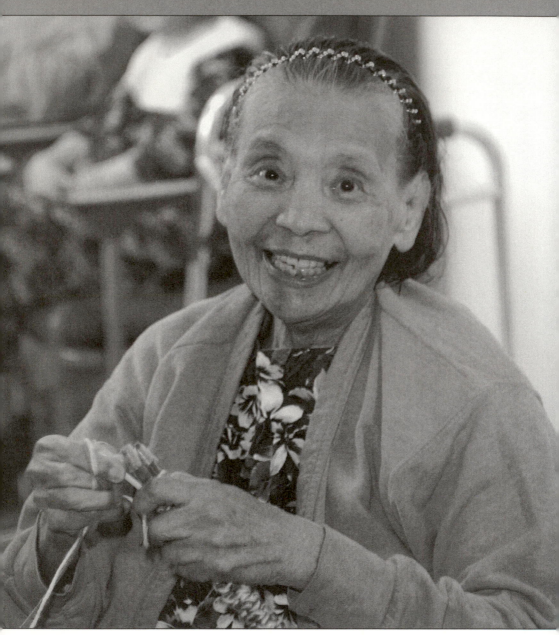

Older Vietnamese Americans

Doorway Thoughts
Although the population from Vietnam is relatively new in North America, it is very diverse in education, religion, degree of acculturation to the new culture, and most other health-related characteristics. It is very important for clinicians caring for older Vietnamese Americans not to make assumptions about individual patients' backgrounds.

Preferred Cultural Terms
The preferred term for patients' cultural and ethnic identity is *Vietnamese Americans* or *Vietnamese people*. *Refugees* or *boat people* may be considered offensive by some elders.

Formality of Address
In formal settings older adults usually expect to be addressed by title (e.g., Mr. or Mrs.) plus the family name, which may be listed first when the name is given. For example, in the name Nguyen Tran, the family name is Nguyen (pronounced "nwin") and the preferred form of address would be Mr. Nguyen. In informal settings, title plus given name may be preferred: Mr. Tran. It is acceptable to ask the elderly Vietnamese patient what his or her preference is for being addressed.

Language and Literacy
Most Vietnamese elders currently living in North America were born in Vietnam, and their first language is most likely Vietnamese. Vietnam is distinctly divided both culturally and socially into three separate regions: Bac (or North), Trung (or Central), and Nam (or South). Regional differences are reflected in the Vietnamese language. The primary language for all three regions is Vietnamese, but differences in pronunciation and intonation distinguish people from the different regions. Many Vietnamese also speak French, English, or one of the Chinese languages. Those who immigrated

between 1975 and 1977 are more likely to speak English, especially those who worked for the U.S. armed forces. Those who came in later waves may have less fluency in English, especially if they were from farming or fishing families.

Respectful Nonverbal Communication

Many Vietnamese family members expect that the elderly person will be shown respect because of the prestige the elders traditionally have in Vietnamese society. Respect is usually shown by:

- Avoiding direct eye contact, especially with elders and other persons of higher status, which may include health care providers
- A slight bow when greeting someone
- Using both hands when giving something to someone else
- Keeping one's arms crossed or hands folded in front

Many older Vietnamese persons, especially those who are less acculturated, may be unfamiliar with the practice of shaking hands and may avoid doing so. Shaking hands with a woman may be considered inappropriate unless she offers her hand first.

Interpersonal space in conversation with a Vietnamese person may be slightly more distant, but sometimes more close, than is common in North America. Raising one's voice, pointing, or openly expressing emotion may be considered disrespectful or in bad taste, depending on the region from which the older person originated in Vietnam. As with language speech patterns, each of the three geographical regions of Vietnam is said to have its own interactional style. Northern and Central Vietnamese are known for being more formal and reserved, and Southerners have a reputation for being less so. As with any generalization, it is always a good idea to observe an individual's interactions and seek clarification if needed.

> *Raising one's voice, pointing, or openly expressing emotion may be considered disrespectful or in bad taste.*

History of Traumatic Experiences

The older Vietnamese patient may have been a refugee or may be a survivor of violence. Are family members missing or dead? Has the patient or family members been tortured or imprisoned?

Common experiences reported by older Vietnamese Americans include:

- Trauma associated with the hasty and chaotic evacuation during the fall of Saigon. Many had less than 24 hours to prepare.
- Repression and persecution under the Communist rule in Vietnam after 1975
- Hunger and starvation during the escape from Vietnam in small, overcrowded, unseaworthy boats
- Months or years in overcrowded refugee camps in Thailand or other Asian countries
- Severe discrimination in the United States in relation to economic competition

Such experiences could negatively affect the health care encounter without the clinician's knowledge unless relevant questions are included among standard questions about the patient's history.

Immigration Status

Most of the first wave of Vietnamese came to the United States as refugees, a status that provided more service benefits than were provided for those who came later as legal immigrants.

Degree of Acculturation

The range of acculturation of older Vietnamese Americans is very broad. Some are perfectly comfortable in North American society, and others are dependent on younger family members when they are outside of the Vietnamese American community. A person's language ability is probably the best single indicator of the level of acculturation.

Vietnamese immigrants who came shortly after the fall of Saigon (1975–1977) were generally well educated, from urban and Catholic backgrounds. Later waves were more heterogeneous, including those who were less well educated and less familiar with English and with Western thought. Groups immigrating in 1979 included people who had spent time in refugee camps and were less healthy. Many Vietnamese elderly persons continue to arrive from Vietnam as "followers of children" in family reunification programs.

Tradition and Health Beliefs

Many Vietnamese Americans hold health beliefs that resemble mainstream Western biomedical views but that also include traditional Asian beliefs about healing. Before immigrating to North

America, most Vietnamese were influenced by classical Chinese beliefs in the need for balance between *yin* and *yang* (also known as *hot* and *cold*). In addition, French medical practices influenced Vietnam during the period of French occupation. Other traditions include beliefs in both natural and supernatural causes of illness, such as the violation of a religious taboo.

> It is important not to confuse marks caused by cupping or coin rubbing with signs of elder abuse.

Illness is sometimes attributed to "catching bad wind." This is often treated by cupping (burning a candle in a glass cup and placing the cup on the skin) or coining (using an oiled coin to rub the chest or back in parallel lines), which may produce superficial abrasions. It is important not to confuse such lesions with signs of elder abuse.

Vietnamese immigrants who have experienced health care in Vietnam commonly expect shots for treatment, as they are frequently used in present-day Vietnam. Clinicians may also want to provide education regarding the use of antibiotics, which are too often stored and shared in the mistaken belief that they will cure common ailments.

Culture-Specific Health Risks
In addition to the health risks of all older Americans, older Vietnamese immigrants have been found to be at increased risk for the following conditions:

Cancer
Vietnamese women have the highest cervical cancer rates reported in the United States, and they are also at higher risk for stomach and thyroid cancers. Vietnamese men have excess rates for nasopharynx, liver, and stomach cancers.

Cardiovascular and Diabetes Risk Factors
Vietnamese men have been found to have high rates of smoking (35% to 54%), which increases their risk of heart disease and stroke. One study found higher rates of insulin resistance among Vietnamese with hypertension, in spite of very slight or no excess weight.

Hepatitis B
More than 80% of Vietnamese elders have been exposed to hepatitis B; one study found that 14% were chronic carriers.

Other Conditions

Other conditions that have been found to be more common among Vietnamese Americans are depression and ova parasites.

Approaches to Decision Making

The family is the most important decision-making unit in traditional Vietnamese culture. Most sources indicate that the responsibility for health care decisions for Vietnamese elders tends to reside with younger family members, although some older Vietnamese Americans may prefer to make their own decisions. One approach would be to ask the older patients whom they would choose to make their health care decisions.

Because family members are often involved in the health care issues and decision making of the older Vietnamese person, it is important to keep family members informed of the patient's health status and needs. Even though many Vietnamese patients and their families will defer to the physician's knowledge and perceived authority, it is nevertheless good practice to include both the older person and his or her family in decisions regarding health and health care.

> *For Vietnamese elders, nodding the head may show courtesy rather than understanding or consent.*

Disclosure and Consent

Simple explanations are advisable. For Vietnamese elders, nodding the head may show courtesy rather than understanding or consent.

Most studies have found that most, but not all, Vietnamese family members do not want the patient to be told that he or she has a serious or terminal illness. Their intention is to prevent additional stress, but this may make obtaining informed consent difficult. Consulting with a designated family spokesperson before giving bad news to an older patient is advisable. It is also advisable to establish preferences regarding information disclosure directly with older Vietnamese patients well in advance of urgent health situations.

Gender Issues

Traditional Vietnamese society is patriarchal, with women assuming the homemaking and caregiving functions. However, many elderly women have had business experience, possibly while in Vietnam. In North America, it is quite common for women to be employed, although preference is most often still given to men in the decision-making role. Women are expected to be the primary caregivers if a parent or any other family member becomes ill.

End-of-Life Decision Making and Care Intensity

The attitudes toward end-of-life issues among Vietnamese immigrants in North America are influenced by spiritual beliefs that are predominantly linked to Catholicism or Buddhism. Nevertheless, beliefs associated with Confucianism and Taoism are not uncommon. Reverence for ancestors and the use of home altars where homage is paid to family ancestors are very common among Vietnamese families.

Studies conducted in the United States report several spiritually based Vietnamese beliefs that are likely to affect decisions at the end of life. These include:

- An aversion to dying in the hospital because of the belief that souls of those who die outside the home wander with no place to rest
- The perception that consenting to end-of-life support for a terminally ill parent contributes to the parent's death and is an insult to one's ancestors
- Buddhist beliefs in karma that interpret difficult deaths as punishment for bad deeds in former lives by the dying person or another family member
- Resistance to organ donation

It is not uncommon among Vietnamese elders to make preparations for death, including putting aside money to pay for burial, choosing a burial site with a favorable orientation, buying a coffin, and buying burial clothes long before they are actually needed. In a study conducted in Hawaii, Vietnamese participants said that common preparations for death also included praying a great deal and preparing wills for distribution of property.

Preferences regarding intensity of care among Vietnamese Americans are not addressed in the published literature.

Use of Advance Directives

Active end-of-life care planning is an unfamiliar undertaking for most Vietnamese families. A study conducted in Hawaii reported that few Vietnamese elders were aware of their options with regard to advance directives. Questions regarding issues related to do-not-resuscitate orders or removal of feeding tubes have usually not been pondered.

| CASE STUDY **1** | **Solving the Headache Puzzle** |

Objectives
1. Examine the historical antecedents and explanatory models of symptoms brought to the clinical setting by older Vietnamese patients.
2. Discuss the potential impact of the historical experience of trauma on the health of older Vietnamese individuals.

Dr. Victoria Wilson is a family physician who completed a fellowship in geriatrics 3 years ago and is practicing in a busy outpatient clinic in a large metropolitan city.

Mr. Tran is a 72-year-old Vietnamese man who has lived in the United States for 14 years. He lives with his son, his son's wife, and their two children. He speaks little English and seldom interacts with anyone outside of the Vietnamese American community.

Mr. Tran came to the clinic as a new patient. He arrived with his daughter-in-law, who attempted to interpret for him with clinic personnel, but her English was not easy for the clerk to understand. When the medical assistant attempted to call Mr. Tran into the exam room based on the name that was on the chart, he did not respond until she walked over to stand in front of him and motioned for him and his daughter-in-law to follow her.

During the introductions, Dr. Wilson discovered that Mr. Tran's name was recorded incorrectly on the chart. His family name, Tran, was written first and assumed to be his given name. She confirmed that he preferred to be called Mr. Tran and corrected the chart. After repeated attempts to interview him for his chief complaint using his daughter-in-law to interpret, Dr. Wilson felt that she did not have enough accurate information to suggest an intervention, so she asked for a Vietnamese interpreter, only to find one was not available for the clinic. She then asked to be connected to the telephone interpreter service, which was completed after a short delay.

When Dr. Wilson was finally able to talk with Mr. Tran through an interpreter on the phone, he seemed reluctant to say much. She did find out by talking both with him and his daughter-in-law through the phone service that he had been having severe headaches, many times so severe that he became dizzy. He also complained of sleepless nights and severe fatigue. He denied having a history of significant illnesses and said he was not taking any medications. Since Mr. Tran was only scheduled for a short appointment, and so much time had been taken up with trying to solve the problems with interpretation, the physician decided to prescribe a nonsteroidal anti-inflammatory for the headaches and schedule a follow-up appointment in a week to take a more complete history. She also ordered some preliminary laboratory tests.

Mr. Tran arrived on schedule for his follow-up appointment, again with his daughter-in-law. This time Dr. Wilson had arranged for a professional Vietnamese interpreter to be present for the appointment. Although the interpreter was from central Vietnam and spoke that dialect, and Mr. Tran was from the southern part of the country that uses a different pronunciation, they were able to understand each other most of the time. This time, Mr. Tran seemed more comfortable talking and was responsive to the questions posed to him. The lab reports were in the normal range.

Mr. Tran's history revealed that he had been an officer in the South Vietnamese army during the Vietnam War. After the war, he had been taken prisoner and sent to reeducation camps by the communists, where he had been tortured. After 3 years he was released. He, his wife, their son, and their daughter-in-law had then managed to escape to Thailand where they were in a refugee camp for 5 years. During that time, his wife became very ill and died. Finally he and his son's family were allowed to come as refugees to the United States. His son initially found work as a fisherman, but then studied English and computers and obtained a job as a computer programmer. Mr. Tran felt he was too old to learn the skills necessary to get a job in the United States. He spends most of his time at home. He sometimes watches his two young grandchildren when his daughter-in-law goes shopping. He has three or four older Vietnamese men friends he gets together with two or three times a week at a local Vietnamese restaurant where they reminisce about their days in Vietnam. His affect seemed flat as he talked about his current life, and he seemed close to tears as he described his experiences in the reeducation and refugee camps, especially the loss of his wife.

Mr. Tran's headaches began about 10 years ago and have been getting increasingly more severe. He reported having headaches two or three times a week on average with no apparent trigger. He has taken over-the-counter medications obtained by his son without much relief. He has also tried Chinese herbal medications because he thought the symptoms might be related to having excess "hot" in his body. He has also tried coining to release excess "wind." Neither of these remedies has been effective for very long. He reported that the nonsteroidal anti-inflammatory medicine that Dr. Wilson prescribed helped a little, but he still has the headaches and feels dizzy.

When Dr. Wilson inquired about the sleeplessness Mr. Tran had complained about, he reported that he frequently has sleepless nights. When he does sleep, he often is awakened by nightmares.

Dr. Wilson ordered an MRI to rule out a brain tumor, prescribed a mild sedative to assist with Mr. Tran's sleep, and made another appointment to see him in 2 weeks.

Results of the MRI showed no brain abnormalities.

Questions:

1. How did availability of language interpretation change care for Mr. Tran? Include issues of clinical accuracy, client-provider relationship, and client satisfaction in your answer.
2. How could the delays and inefficiencies related to language in the clinic be reduced?
3. What do you think the possible causes are for Mr. Tran's headaches?
4. Which explanatory models does Mr. Tran use to explain his symptoms?
5. Dr. Wilson suspects post traumatic stress disorder (PTSD). How could she approach assisting Mr. Tran?

In the next appointment, Dr. Wilson decided to try to explore Mr. Tran's explanatory models of his condition that she had learned about in Continuing Medical Education courses on ethnogeriatrics, including his perception of what caused the headaches and sleeplessness. Through the interpreter, she learned that he thought that his headaches and dizziness were caused by "thinking too much." When she pursued what he might have been thinking about, he talked about the torture he experienced in the reeducation camps, the terrible conditions in the refugee camps, his wife's illness and death, and the loss of other friends and family members in the war and postwar chaos in Vietnam. She also found out that his nightmares frequently had the same content.

With this information, Dr. Wilson was convinced that Mr. Tran might profit from post traumatic stress therapy. She prescribed a low dose of a recommended antidepressant for older adults, but felt that it was more important that he have access to appropriate psychotherapy. Because the therapists she knew did not speak Vietnamese, and because she realized that psychotherapy through an interpreter would be very difficult, she was at a loss to know where to turn. She asked the interpreter who was working with her if he knew any Vietnamese psychotherapists, and he suggested calling the Vietnamese senior center run by Catholic Charities. Through that contact, Dr. Wilson found a mental health clinic with Vietnamese therapists and made the referral.

Initially, Mr. Tran and his daughter-in-law were reluctant for him to see a therapist, maintaining through the interpreter that he was not "crazy." Dr. Wilson asked him what would be important to make him comfortable in seeing a therapist to help with his "thinking too much." His daughter-in-law stressed the importance of showing him appropriate respect as an elder to make him feel comfortable, which he had not felt initially in his interaction with the medical clinic until he communicated through the interpreter who used the appropriate language and gestures to confer respect. After considerable discussion and reassurance that Dr. Wilson would communicate his concerns to the therapist, he agreed to go to the mental health clinic.

| CASE STUDY **2** | **One Little Vietnamese Lady in a Big American Nursing Home** |

Objectives
1. Analyze factors influencing Vietnamese family members' decisions on end-of-life care.
2. Develop culturally sensitive strategies to meet the special needs of Vietnamese elders living in long-term care facilities.

The setting is a 99-bed for-profit nursing home in a large city in the American midwest. Dr. Finley, the medical director, is an internist with extensive experience in long-term care. No nurse practitioners are available on staff in this nursing home.

Dr. Finley was requested to assume the care of Mrs. Nguyen, an 85-year-old Vietnamese woman who was recently admitted to the nursing home. Her Vietnamese physician who had been her primary care provider does not follow patients in nursing homes.

When Dr. Finley reviewed her chart, he found that Mrs. Nguyen was a monolingual Vietnamese-speaking elder with severe dementia. He visited her bedside and found a small woman who was nonresponsive to him and was mumbling something he did not understand. He performed a preliminary physical examination with no remarkable findings. He realized he would not be able to administer a mini-mental exam or perform any other assessments without assistance from someone who speaks Vietnamese.

Dr. Finley asked the nursing home administrator for assistance with language interpreting and found that there were no Vietnamese-speaking staff. Because Mrs. Nguyen was the only resident who spoke Vietnamese, the nursing home could not afford to pay for an interpreter and asked him to use her family members. Dr. Finley reviewed the nursing and dietitian assessment notes and found that she was free of skin breakdown and had evidently been well cared for at home before admission. She had lost 3 pounds since being admitted 10 days ago and was refusing to eat or take liquid nutritional supplements. Nursing staff were concerned that pressure sores would develop if her nutritional status did not improve.

According to the social work notes, Mrs. Nguyen's only family member listed was her daughter, Kim Nguyen, who lived nearby and visited her mother daily. Dr. Finley asked to have an appointment made to talk with the daughter in hopes that he could obtain assistance with assessments and information on the patient's history.

Ms. Kim Nguyen (Kim) met Dr. Finley at the appointed time in her mother's room. She was a well-groomed Vietnamese woman who appeared to be in her late 50s. She spoke in broken, but understandable, English. With her assistance, Dr. Finley asked Mrs. Nguyen about her pain level and some basic orientation and memory questions. He realized that many of the formal questions on the mini-mental state exam would be useless because they might not be relevant to her experience or it would be impossible for the questions to be translated appropriately (e.g., "no ifs, ands, or buts"). She was able to respond to some simple commands and yes-or-no questions, but appeared to be in the advanced stages of dementia. She obviously recognized her daughter, but was not able to say who she was.

On being questioned about her mother's nutritional status, the daughter indicated that the only foods her mother would eat were traditional Vietnamese dishes. The liquid supplements the staff tried to give her were foreign to her tastes.

On their second meeting, Dr. Finley cautiously approached the subject of Do Not Resuscitate (DNR) orders and advance directives for her mother with Kim. Her adamant response was that she wanted everything done to extend her mother's life as long as possible, including a feeding tube if her mother were no longer able to swallow. In exploring these issues, the following history emerged.

Mrs. Nguyen had been widowed for 20 years. She began showing signs of disorientation and memory loss while she was still living in Vietnam, where Kim lived nearby and worked in a clothing shop. Two of Mrs. Nguyen's older sons had immigrated to the United States in the late 1980s. When Mrs. Nguyen became too impaired to live alone, the oldest son sponsored Kim and their mother to join him and his family in the United States. When they arrived, the family decided that Kim would continue to live with and care for her mother with some financial help from her brothers because neither of the brothers' homes was large enough to accommodate Kim and their mother. The assistance they could afford, however, was not sufficient to pay all their expenses, so Kim was forced to take a job in a restaurant.

As her mother's dementia progressed, it became increasingly difficult to care for her adequately alone. Mrs. Nguyen began to wander outside the house while Kim was at work and became incontinent of urine and feces. Kim consulted her Vietnamese physician and was told that her mother's condition was a result of her "brain going flat," a common untreatable condition of old age. When Kim talked to her brothers about the problems she was having, they felt it was extremely important for their mother to be cared for by family members, but no one was able to assist enough to have someone with Mrs. Nguyen all the time.

Kim began losing weight and having frequent asthma attacks. She felt increasingly desperate about her situation and decided to talk with her priest about her options. He suggested she consider placing her mother in a nursing home. When Kim talked to them, both her brothers were strongly opposed to considering a nursing home and felt it was not the Vietnamese way of honoring one's elders and ancestors, so she felt very guilty even considering it. When it became obvious to all that Kim would not be able to continue alone with her mother's need for round-the-clock care because of her own declining health, the oldest brother, who had legal responsibility for their mother as her sponsor, reluctantly agreed to consider a placement. In prayer with her priest and members of her church, Kim decided that if her mother was accepted by the nursing home, it would be a signal that it would be God's will that she should go.

In conversation with Dr. Finley, Kim continually made reference to the good 24-hour care her mother received in the nursing home, much better than she could provide because she at least had to sleep and go shopping for food. It was clear to Dr. Finley that Kim was still struggling with the heavy guilt she felt in placing her mother and needed to find rationalizations for her action.

Questions:

1. What culturally sensitive strategies could be implemented to increase Mrs. Nguyen's nutritional intake?
2. What cultural and historical factors are influencing the decisions Kim is making about DNR orders and advance directives?
3. How should Dr. Finley approach the negotiation of end-of-life decisions with Mrs. Nguyen?

In team conference, the staff decides to try to develop some innovative strategies to improve Mrs. Nguyen's nutritional status. The dietitian met with Kim to get information about Mrs. Nguyen's food preferences and ways to prepare food she might eat. Kim agreed to try to bring a traditional Vietnamese meal for her mother's evening meal every day. For the other meals, the dietitian agreed to prepare a rice dish. She would research Vietnamese sauces that would be available from Vietnamese grocery stores or resources on international foods and offer them to Mrs. Nguyen using Kim's suggestions for her preferences.

Dr. Finley suggested that the staff ask the local Vietnamese priest to come to a staff meeting to help them understand the issues related to filial piety in the Vietnamese culture. They would also ask him to help them talk with Kim about the DNR orders and advance directives.

Jane Uyen Tran, MSW
Gwen Yeo, PhD

References

Braun KL, Browne CV. Perceptions of dementia, caregiving, and help seeking among Asian and Pacific Islander Americans. *Health Soc Work* 1998; 23(4):262–274.

Braun KL, Nichols R. Cultural issues in death and dying. *Hawaii Med J* 1996;55(12):260–264.

Calhoun MA. Providing health care to Vietnamese in America: what practitioners need to know. *Home Healthc Nurse* 1986;4(5):14–22.

Nowak TT. Vietnamese Americans. In Purnell LD, Paulanka BJ, eds. *Transcultural Health Care: A Culturally Competent Approach*. Philadelphia: F. A. Davis; 1998.

Ta M, Chung C. Death and dying: a Vietnamese cultural perspective. In: Parry JK, ed. *Social Work Practice with the Terminally Ill: A Transcultural Perspective*. Springfield, IL: Charles C. Thomas; 1990.

Yee, BWK. Health and health care of Southeast Asian American elders: Vietnamese, Cambodian, Hmong, and Laotian elders. In: Yeo G, ed. *Ethnic Specific Modules of the Curriculum in Ethnogeriatrics*. Stanford, CA: Stanford Geriatric Education Center; 2002. (Available at http://www.stanford.edu/group/ethnoger)

Yeo G. Ethical considerations in Asian and Pacific Island elders. *Clin Geriatr Med* 1995;11(1):139–151.

Yeo G, Hikoyeda N. Asians and Pacific Islanders in the United States. In Braun KL, Pietsch JH, Blanchette PL, eds. *Cultural Issues in End-of-Life Decision Making*. Thousand Oaks, CA: Sage Publications; 2000.

Yeo G, Hikoyeda N, McBride M, et al. *Cohort Analysis as a Tool in Ethnogeriatrics: Historical Profiles of Elders from Eight Ethnic Populations in the United States*. Stanford GEC Working Paper #12. Stanford, CA: Stanford Geriatric Education Center; 1998.

Yeo G, Tran JNU, Hikoyeda N, et al. Concepts of dementia among Vietnamese American caregivers. *J Gerontol Soc Work* 2001;36(1/2):131–152.

CHAPTER 6

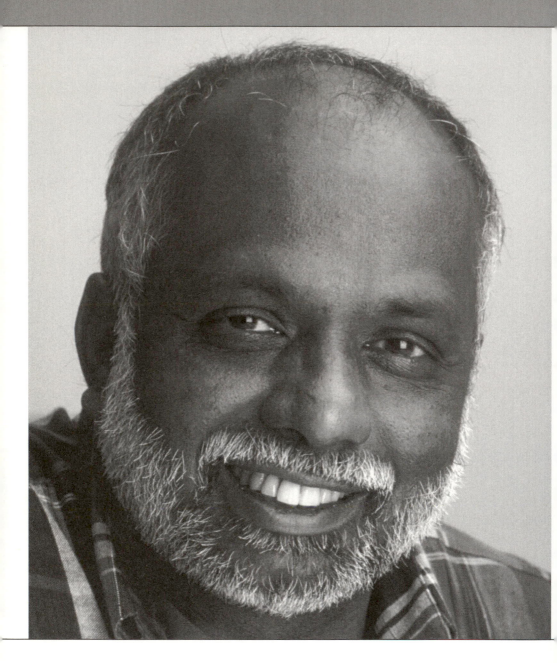

Older Asian Indian Americans

Doorway Thoughts

The concept of respect is extremely important to traditional Asian Indians. Respect focuses on the moral obligation to honor the essential worth of every individual. This obligation is considered to be even more important when one is dealing with an older person. In India, old age is synonymous with wisdom.

Preferred Cultural Terms

There is a certain ambiguity (especially in North America) associated with the term *Indian*. It is often confused with the terms *American Indian* and *Native American*, which are commonly used to denote the indigenous peoples in the United States. The term *Native American* is confusing because anyone born in the Americas can be referred to as a "native American," and there are numerous second-generation Asian Indians who would belong to this cohort. The term *American Indian* can also be confusing, as this term can denote India-born immigrants who become American citizens by naturalization. Therefore, it is preferable to use the term *Asian Indians* to denote peoples of (Asian) Indian origins, while remembering that this is not necessarily a homogeneous population.

Formality of Address

Asian Indian elders expect respectful and deferential treatment as their due. The clinician who clearly communicates an attitude of respect for an Asian Indian elder is more likely to establish rapport with the patient. Patients should be addressed warmly but formally (e.g., Mr. or Mrs.) until they give permission to use their first names, if they ever do.

The clinician who clearly communicates an attitude of respect for an Asian Indian elder is more likely to establish rapport with the patient.

Language and Literacy

Most Asian Indian immigrants are well educated, and many are well-qualified professionals. Over 85% of Indians in the United States have graduated from high school, over 65% have college degrees, and approximately 43% have graduate or professional degrees.

Effective Communication

The clinician needs to be self-assured while respecting personal boundaries: Asian Indian elders are socialized in an ancient system of patriarchal medicine in which the physician takes control and makes most decisions. Even though Asian Indians in the United States are adapting to a medical system in which the patient is often viewed and treated as the customer, they are likely to perceive any expression of uncertainty, even if appropriate, as ineptness and lack of medical competence. For example, saying "Mr. Patel, I think that, given your clinical picture, what you have is probably a lung cancer; I could be wrong about this, but probably not. . . ." would not be as advisable as saying "Mr. Patel, I am sorry, but I have some bad news for you. Given all the test results, I think that you have a lung cancer." At the same time, expecting Asian Indian elders to be more involved in medical decision making than they want to be is not advisable.

It may be useful to remember that Asian Indians are more relation oriented than task oriented. The role of the clinician as a healer is greatly respected in India, and Asian Indian elders will often treat the physician with deferential respect. This may mean that they will not voice issues that they perceive as being less important on the physician's agenda. It is important, therefore, to probe subtly to identify issues that are not being addressed.

Asian Indians belong to a culture that values the past and may even believe that the future is determined by the actions in the past. Elders do respect the American concept of punctuality and are seldom late for health care appointments, but the concept of time in India is more loosely structured and not quite as rigid as in the United States. In contrast to the Western linear concept of time, where seconds add up to minutes and minutes to hours, to the Asian Indian time is nonlinear and even viewed as cyclical, with the soul repeatedly undergoing the birth-death cycle. Relationships are valued more than rigid schedules, and Indian elders may therefore seem to focus on trivial minutiae of their medical care. An abrupt termination of the clinical encounter in deference to punctuality may be perceived as rude or disrespectful. Explaining to the patient that you are running late and that other patients are waiting will go a long way to placate the irate elder who is upset at what he or she sees as the premature termination of the medical visit.

History of Immigration and Acculturation

The earliest record of an Indian traveling to the United States is that of a young Indian man from south India who may have visited Massachusetts in 1790. American trade with India during the early years of the Republic brought young Indians to work on the wharves in New England. Americans' interest in Eastern culture and spirituality culminated in the 19th century in the appearance of Swami Vivekananda, the renowned Hindu yogi, when he addressed the World Parliament of Religions in Chicago in 1893. In the early 1900s a number of Indians from Punjab migrated to the western United States to take jobs in the Pacific Northwest working for lumber mills and all along the Pacific coast working on the railroads.

The "Barred Zone Act" of 1917 put a stop to Indian immigration until a bill allowing Indian naturalization and immigration was finally passed in July 1946. The number of Indians coming annually to the United States until 1965 remained in the hundreds. With the Immigration Act of 1965, Indian immigration increased dramatically, with tens of thousands coming each year in the 1980s and 1990s.

Tradition and Health Beliefs

Asian Indian elders who immigrated to the United States late in life may still be more wedded to traditional Indian healing practices (e.g., Ayurveda, Unani). In contrast, elders who have spent the majority of their adult lives in the United States are more prone to embrace modern biomedicine.

Professionals in biomedicine command enormous respect, prestige, and admiration among Indians. Asian Indians elders may defer to their physicians even for simple decisions and so may ask many trivial questions about their medicines

Asian Indian elders may ask many questions about their medicines and diet.

and diet. Although this may be time consuming for the busy practitioner, it is the elder's way of showing respect for the clinician and should be viewed as such. Overall, Asian Indian elders willingly submit to laboratory tests and medical or surgical procedures as needed.

Many Indians wear religious paraphernalia; examples include special clothing (*tupi*, a religious cap worn by Moslems), sacred ornaments (*mangalsutra*, a necklace worn by married Hindu women), sacred threads around the body (worn by Hindu males), or amulets (*kara*, a steel bracelet worn by Sikh men who have undergone the Amrit ceremony or baptism). These are considered sacred and should never be removed or cut without the consent of the patient or a family member.

Many Asian Indians practice Hinduism or Sikhism and believe in reincarnation, that is, that every living being has multiple lives and goes through the cycle of birth and death multiple times. The word *karma* (from the Sanskrit root *kri* meaning "to do") can be understood to denote the fruit of actions. One's actions (good or bad) during previous lives are thought to influence the events of future lives to come. Asian Indian elders therefore may believe that illnesses are the result of bad karma from the past lives and so may be less inclined to adhere to biomedical regimens, as they may feel that these interventions are powerless in the face of karma. Also, the belief in reincarnation may strongly influence the way they perceive and find meaning in their life and death. Moslems also believe that bad actions (not necessarily from past lives) result in illnesses and that the illness washes away the sins.

Ayurveda, the ancient Indian science of healing, has been practiced for almost 5,000 years. Ayurveda describes three fundamental universal energies that regulate all natural processes on both the macrocosmic and microcosmic levels. These three energy systems are known as the *tridosha* and consist of *pitha* (bile), *vatha* (wind, air), and *kapha* (phlegm). In a healthy person these three driving forces are perfectly balanced. Any disequilibrium between these three energies, which might be excess (*vrddhi*) or deficiency (*ksaya*), manifests as a sign or symptom of disease. Ayurvedic principles have been in practice for so long that they have been absorbed into everyday thought and practice. Asian Indians may follow these principles unconsciously. Some common beliefs based on these principles include the conviction that milk and bananas should not be eaten together, and that drinking warm water promotes health and drinking cold water makes the body vulnerable to illness.

Asian Indian patients may also be taking ayurvedic herbs and alternative medicines even while on allopathic treatment. The clinician should remember to routinely inquire about such practices. In addition, Asian Indian elders, especially those who come from rural areas, may believe that certain diseases are caused by evil spirits and so practice rituals to cleanse the possessed individual.

Upwas, or fasting, is a common practice among the elderly of India, especially the women. *Upwas* is thought to spiritually strengthen the person and also bring good luck to the family. Persons observing *upwas* may eat just fruits and, in extreme cases, some will observe a complete fast and may not even drink water. This practice may have several health implications, especially for those with diabetes mellitus or hypovolemia and orthostatic hypotension.

Dil udas hona is the term for the "blues" in the Hindi, Urdu, Punjabi, and Gujarati languages. Having the blues may be thought to be due to bad karma, possibily making depressed patients resistant to or apathetic about the idea of medical interventions.

Asian Indians believe that the outcomes of a deed may be influenced by the time when it was done, that is, that actions undertaken during inauspicious times are unlikely to succeed. There are spells of such inauspicious times every day (*rahukaala*). There are also auspicious days and inauspicious days, as determined by the Indian lunar calendar. Asian Indian elders often follow this calendar and may be very hesitant about having surgeries or procedures during inauspicious times.

> *Having the "blues" may be thought to be due to bad karma, so depressed patients may be resistant to or apathetic about the idea of medical interventions.*

Culture-Specific Health Risks

Multiple studies have shown that Asian Indian elders have a high risk for coronary artery disease and diabetes mellitus. Increased visceral fat is related to dyslipidemia and increased incidence of insulin resistance and may account for the increased prevalence of diabetes mellitus and cardiovascular disease among Asian Indians.

Asian Indians from the Indian subcontinent have low rates of breast cancer, but one study of breast cancer risk factors in Indian and Pakistani premenopausal women living in the United States that compared them with their American counterparts showed that the risk factors were determined more by environmental factors than by ethnicity.

As many elders have the habit of chewing *pan* (tobacco with spices), they are at increased risk for oral submucosal fibrosis.

Elderly migrants who are dependent on their families financially and who are also living in relative social isolation resulting from their immigrant status may experience profound loneliness and diminished self-esteem, resulting in depression.

Approaches to Decision Making

Western concepts of autonomy and surrogate decision making are alien to the Asian Indian culture. Indian culture tends to emphasize interconnectedness and downplay individualism. A person thinks of herself or himself as a part of the family unit, and important decisions are made after consulting with the family. The "family" could be the nuclear family, or it could include members of the extended family. In some cases, close family friends are treated as family and will also be involved in the decision-making process. If there is a medical professional within the family, he or she will be called upon to interpret the illness situation, and the family may even ask the medical relative to call the physician involved and to serve as a liaison with the health care system for the patient and family.

Disclosure and Consent

"Doctor, please do not tell my grandfather that he has cancer and that he is dying." This is not an uncommon request among Asian Indians. The ill Asian Indian individual may defer decision making to his or her family. Some Asian Indians believe that voicing thoughts about death and dying will make it happen. Others believe that the loved one who is told that he or she has cancer will lose the will to live and therefore die sooner.

When faced with this situation, the clinician should verify that the patient is comfortable with letting the family make his or her health care decisions. Saying something like "Mr. Patel, I am told that you prefer to let your sons make all health care decisions for you and that you would prefer not to know your diagnosis. Is this correct?" will help confirm the patient's stance. If the patient prefers not to know about his or her medical condition, this preference should be respected. Autonomy is the right to choose, and patients have the right to choose to remain ignorant of their diagnosis.

Gender Issues

Usually, Asian Indian elders are more comfortable with same-sex providers. The concept of *shrm,* or modesty, is highly valued in the Indian society. Elderly women may be soft-spoken (another trait that is admired) and not advocate for themselves. Out of modesty and shyness or deference to the male accompanying them, they may not voice personal issues (both of physical or psychosocial nature), and they may choose to suffer in silence or assent without agreeing. It is important to talk to the patient confidentially to elicit her preferences. Establishing a bond with patients over time and thus gaining their trust is clinically valuable, as Asian Indian elders are more likely to seek help from those with whom they have rapport.

End-of-Life Decision Making and Care Intensity

Asian Indian elders usually prefer to die peacefully at home surrounded by their loved ones. If they die in the hospital, there is often a strong preference that care be given by same-sex nursing staff.

Asian Indian women may not voice personal issues and may choose to suffer in silence or assent without agreeing.

This is especially true when dealing with the dead body. Asian Indians have extensive death rituals, which vary tremendously among religions and sects, and so it is important to gently inquire about these matters from the patient's relatives in order to avoid cultural faux pas.

Use of Advance Directives

Active end-of-life care planning is an unfamiliar concept to most Asian Indian elders. Physicians who have these discussions should remember that the elders may be reluctant to participate in these discussions, as they may believe that talking about death could make it a reality. Or worse, the elder may believe that the physician is subtly implying that he or she has a serious illness and is dying. Great tact and sensitivity are called for when having these discussions. Ensure that you have adequate time and that the patient's family is present.

| CASE STUDY **1** | **Medication Adherence and the Ayurvedic Herb** |

Objectives

1. Discuss how the communication style of Asian Indian American elders may reveal their attitudes toward physicians.
2. Understand Asian Indian American migration history as it pertains to access to health care.

You are a primary care physician working in a busy urban primary care clinic. It is a hot Friday afternoon, you have had a very busy day with several "drop-ins," and you are tired and somewhat distracted. Before you can start your long-awaited weekend, you have to see one last new patient whom you have not seen before. You have his extensive medical record before you. Mr. Patel is a 74-year-old Asian Indian male with a history of long-standing hypertension and diabetes mellitus not well controlled on medications. Three weeks ago, Mr. Patel suffered a small stroke and was hospitalized for 2 days. At the time of discharge, he was noted to have mild weakness of his left arm and leg and slightly slurred speech. He was discharged on the following medications:

- Lisinopril 20 mg q AM
- Glyburide 5 mg BID
- Agranox (aspirin and dipyramidamole) 1 tablet qd
- MVI 1 tablet qd

The discharging physician also instructed the patient to check his blood sugars three times a day and his blood pressure every day.

Mr. Patel's 71-year-old wife is his primary caregiver. They currently live with their eldest daughter, Rani, who is a software engineer, in Sunnyvale, California. Prior to immigrating to the United States (2 years ago), they lived in Gandhinagar, Gujarat. They have two other daughters who are married and live in Texas.

The patient, his wife, and their oldest daughter have arrived. The clinic nurse tells you that Mr. Patel has not been checking his sugars or his blood pressure. In fact, he has not taken any of his discharge medications except for over-the-counter Aspirin 325 mg twice daily. You wonder whether you will need an interpreter, because you are very concerned about Mr. Patel's nonadherence to his discharge instructions.

You inform the family that you will need to request that a Gujarati interpreter join you in the interview in order to best understand Mr. Patel. His daughter and wife, however, request to be present during the interview with the interpreter. You agree and proceed.

When the interpreter arrives, you introduce yourself to Mr. and Mrs. Patel and their daughter and ask Mr. Patel how he is feeling. He states that he is feeling fine, but proceeds to ask you many detailed questions about the relative advantages of a variety of vegetables and fruits in the care of his diabetes.

Question:

1. How might Mr. Patel's detailed questions reflect his culturally based attitudes toward physicians?

You examine Mr. Patel. His blood pressure is 200/104. His glucometer reading in the office is 288 mg/dl. After the examination, you mention to Mr. Patel that his blood pressure is on the high side, and that it would most likely be in better control if he were taking his medications regularly. Rani tell you that the Patels are not eligible for Medicare, and that money for medications is tight now that they have hospital bills to pay. Mr. Patel has been taking ayurvedic herbs instead, because they are more affordable.

Question:

1. How might understanding Mr. Patel's migration history assist in developing appropriate care plans for him in the future?

You take a full migration history from Mr. Patel and then understand why he may be having difficulty with adherence to his medication and glucometer plan. You give the Patels some samples of HCTZ, 12.5 mg daily, from the office, and give them a follow-up prescription for this medication (cost = $8.00/month). You arrange for the representative from a local glucometer distributor to provide Mr. Patel with new glucometer (last year's model) at no charge. You put Mr. Patel on a staggered schedule for glucose checks (i.e., Monday before breakfast, Tuesday before lunch, Wednesday before supper, and Thursday before bedtime).

When Mr. Patel and his family return to your office one month later, they are very pleased with his progress. His function and energy are improved. His blood pressure on exam is 150/85. His glucometer readings for the month indicate that his control is good, but he is running a bit high (approximately 180 mg/dl before breakfast). You increase his evening dose of glyburide and ask him to continue checking his blood sugar until his next return appointment in 3 weeks.

CASE STUDY **2**	**Please Do Not Tell Her**

Objective
1. Discuss Asian Indian American values and attitudes toward end-of-life planning.

Mrs. Reddy is a 78-year-old Asian Indian female who has been admitted to the hospital with lower gastrointestinal bleeding. The patient was brought into the emergency room 2 days ago with a history of dizziness status post a bowel movement during which she passed a large quantity of bright red blood rectally. You admit the patient to your service and stabilize her by transfusing two units of packed red blood cells. The consulting gastroenterologist does a colonoscopy, which reveals a large mass in the descending colon. A biopsy of the mass reveals it to be an adenocarcinoma of the colon. An abdominal computed tomography reveals local metastatic disease as well as extensive hepatic metastases. Mrs. Reddy is a widow and lives with her only son, Pratap, who is her primary caregiver. Pratap, who is very caring and supportive of his mother, specifically requests that you not tell his mother the diagnosis as "she would lose all hope and die."

Question:
1. What cultural values might Pratap be reflecting when he says, "Don't tell my mother her diagnosis, because she will lose all hope"?

You go back to see Mrs. Reddy the next morning and ask her if she would like you to discuss her health information with her directly, or would she prefer that someone else act as her proxy for information and decisions. She tells you that she would like her son to receive all of her information and make her health decisions for her. You agree to this, and continue to communicate with Pratap for updates and decision making.

Two weeks later, she is functionally declining, and you mention to her that she might be more comfortable in facility care rather than returning home. Although usually Mrs. Reddy is very compliant with physician suggestions, she immediately looks very agitated and states, "I am going home with my son!"

Question:
1. How might Mrs. Reddy's cultural values be reflected in her statement, "I am going home with my son"?

You call a family meeting with Pratap and his wife to discuss discharge planning for his mother. He and his wife agree that they very much want to take Mrs. Reddy home, but you sense that they are feeling a bit overwhelmed with her care needs. You invite the home hospice program to attend the meeting. Their nurse clinician, who is originally from Bombay, assures the family that home support and nursing services that are sensitive to Mrs. Reddy's needs, will be provided. The meeting ends with all parties feeling more secure in the plan.

Vyjeyanthi S. Periyakoil, MD

References

Banerji MA, Faridi N, Atluri R, et al. Body composition, visceral fat, leptin, and insulin resistance in Asian Indian men. *J Clin Endocrinol Metab* 1999; 84(1):137–144.

Helweg AW, Helweg UM. *An Immigrant Success Story: East Indians in America.* Philadelphia: University of Pennsylvania Press; 1990.

Jensen JM. *Passage From India: Asian Indian Immigrants in North America.* New Haven, CT: Yale University Press; 1988.

Kalavar JM. *The Asian Indian Elderly in America.* New York: Garland Publishing; 1998.

Kamath SK, Murillo G, Chatterton RT Jr, et al. Breast cancer risk factors in two distinct ethnic groups: Indian and Pakistani vs. American premenopausal women. *Nutr Cancer* 1999;35(1):16–26.

Kulkarni KR, Markovitz JH, Nanda NC, et al. Increased prevalence of smaller and denser LDL particles in Asian Indians. *Arterioscler Thromb Vasc Biol* 1999;19(11):2749–2755.

Lipson JG, Dibble SL, Minarik PA, eds. *Culture and Nursing Care: A Pocket Guide.* San Francisco, CA: UCSF Nursing Press; 1996.

Periyakoil VS, Yeo G. Understanding the term death with dignity and its implications to ethnic elders. Stanford University project unpublished data. (For information or answers to any questions, communicate with the author by e-mail: Vyjeyanthi S Periyakoil [vsperiyakoil@hotmail.com].)

CHAPTER 7

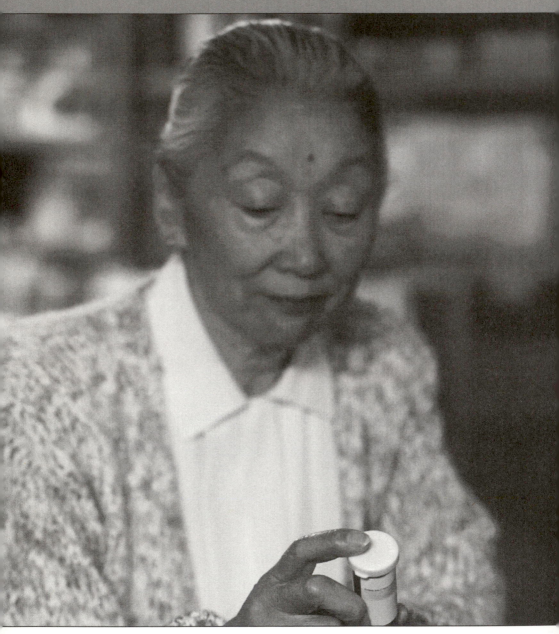

Older Japanese Americans

Doorway Thoughts

Filial piety is a traditionally respected value in Japan. A Confucian virtue with origins in China, it was introduced to Japan in the seventh century. In simple terms, Japanese children were expected not only to honor and respect their parents but also to take care of them in their old age. Although it would seem that all elders would appreciate being treated with courtesy and respect, the Japanese, especially, traditionally hold these as prime virtues. Two other virtues that rank high in traditional Japanese thinking are *omoiyari* ("empathy" or "thoughtfulness") and *kokoro* ("having a good heart"). Thus, the clinician who is empathetic and genuinely caring as well as courteous and respectful will create a basis for an effective clinical relationship with the older Japanese patient.

Preferred Cultural Terms

Generally speaking, as a group, the Japanese Americans should be referred to as *Japanese Americans*. Further defining and addressing the generations (e.g., *issei, nissei,* or *sansei,* as described on page 83) is also acceptable. However, the use of the word *Japs* should be avoided.

Formality of Address

The Japanese language is structured in such a way that the selection and use of words differ, depending on who is speaking to whom. Who is speaking to whom or the reciprocity or nonreciprocity of the speakers is in turn determined by status and group affiliation. When addressing Japanese American elders initially, the use of a formal title (e.g., Mr., Mrs.) with the surname would show respect and thus be appreciated. Another way of addressing the very traditional Japanese-speaking American elder would be to call him or her by surname followed by -*san*, for example, "Suzuki-san." Addressing an elder in this way would come as a welcome and pleasant surprise. Generally speaking, it would be prudent to avoid using first names or addressing an elder as *Grandma* or *Grandpa*.

Language and Literacy

The Japanese Americans are, relatively speaking, an older group in the immigration time line. Most Japanese immigration took place in the early 1900s. As a result, the percentage of Japanese American elders who truly speak only Japanese is low.

Respectful Nonverbal Communication

Among traditional Japanese Americans, the style of communication and discussion is indirect and restrained, rather than direct and forthright, with the aim of avoiding overt confrontation. Thus, a meeting of the family with clinicians in which there is open disagreement, confrontation, and argument as well as debate may be looked upon as *hazukashii* or "an embarrassment" to the family name.

> *Among traditional Japanese Americans, the style of communication aims to avoid overt confrontation.*

History of Immigration

Most of the immigration to the United States from Japan occurred in the late 1800s to early 1900s during the Meiji Era. The governance of Japan by the Shogunate had come to an end, and Japan was emerging from a feudal social structure into a modern one. Sweeping changes were occurring in Japan. Many immigrants in the early 20th century were farmers or laborers; their reasons for immigrating were primarily economic. During this time of sweeping change, it is of interest to note that some traditions remained strong, even with the new Japanese constitution, which had been drawn on Western political models. Traditional views, with ultimate origins in Confucianism, included the belief that society is more important than the individual, and that the patriarchal family with the husband as head is a model for governance of the state. These views can still be seen in very traditional Japanese American families, though less so today than formerly.

A second wave of immigration occurred after World War II, as U.S. servicemen brought Japanese wives to the United States. This generation of immigrants, raised in a different time from the earlier immigrants, held somewhat less traditional views. For those servicemen who brought Japanese wives to the United States, there have been many interesting stories of differing attitudes and conflict among the original Japanese immigrants and the new Japanese wives. The views of the older women were seen as feudal remnants of the Meiji Era.

Degree of Acculturation

There is much diversity among Japanese American elders with respect to the degree with which they embrace traditional Japanese culture and values. The generations are numbered and referred to as *issei* (first), *nissei* (second), *sansei* (third), and so forth. Most of the first generation of Japanese immigrants, the *issei*, immigrated to the United States between the late 1800s and early 1900s. Having been born in Japan, they often held very traditional values and had strong cultural ties with the homeland. The second-generation Japanese Americans, the *nissei*, were raised through the Depression and World War II. They were brought up in two cultural worlds, the American and Japanese. The third generation, the *sansei*, and the fourth generation, the *yonsei*, are the most acculturated to the American ways. Many cannot speak the Japanese language, and marriage outside of the ethnic group is common.

An additional group, the *kibbei*, is the generation of Japanese Americans who were born in the United States but were "sent back" to be raised and educated in Japan. Most of the *kibbei* were born in the 1920s and 1930s. Some were stranded in Japan during World War II.

There is a broad spectrum among Japanese Americans with respect to degree of acculturation. In general, with the passing of generations, many have married outside their ethnic background and have not held onto Japanese traditions and values. In addition, with respect to religion, one will find many Christian Japanese Americans. Japan itself is a dynamic society that seems to be experiencing some shift in traditional values.

Tradition and Health Beliefs

In the traditional Japanese culture, the concept of the gift has played an important role in supporting and maintaining the fabric of society. In addition to events that are defined as gift-giving occasions, such as birth, employment, and marriage, unexpected events, such as an illness (*mimai*) or loss in a natural disaster, are also occasions for giving gifts. In traditional Japan but probably less among Japanese American elders, gifts are also given in midsummer (*chugen*) and at the end of the year (*seibo*). The clinician caring for Japanese American elders may receive gifts if the patient or family feels indebted for care that goes beyond what is customary. For example, a nurse making a home visit may end up receiving a box of candies as a token of appreciation.

In Japan, shoes are traditionally removed at the entrance of the home before entering the door. In a traditional Japanese American home, this custom may be maintained. Thus, it would be courteous for clinicians to offer to remove their shoes when making a home visit or house call.

In a very traditional family, gifts are not usually opened in front of the giver unless permission is asked. If a gift is opened in front of the giver, the wrapping is usually delicately and carefully removed. Generalized and vigorous tearing of the wrapping is avoided.

Traditional medical practice in Japan was heavily influenced by the Chinese concepts of *yin* and *yang* and the flow of energy. The use of medications (often herbal), along with acupuncture, moxibustion, and massage, was aimed at restoring balance between the *yin* and *yang* elements of the body. Moxibustion is the process of placing and burning a small cone composed of mugwort leaves on specific points on the skin.

Generally, aside from the recent resurgence in the use of acupuncture and massage, most Japanese Americans today rely on mainstream Western medicine. With respect to health services, however, very traditional families may be reluctant to actively seek out mental health services early, as there is a general stigma associated with mental illnesses. In addition, there may be a reluctance to report changes in mental status, which raises the possibility of undiagnosed dementia.

Culture-Specific Health Risks

Studies from the Honolulu Heart Program and the Honolulu-Asia Aging Study suggest that vascular dementia among Japanese American men may be higher than it is among white men. Other studies suggest that with increasing adaptation to the Western diet (greater proportions of meat, less roughage), there appears to be an increase in coronary artery disease and colon cancer among Japanese Americans.

Approaches to Decision Making

In a very traditional Japanese family where hierarchical principles are maintained, major decisions are delegated to the oldest male. The oldest son is the decision maker even if there is a daughter older than the son. If the family is very traditional, then there is usually no overt disagreement with the decisions made by the oldest son. However, with the increasing acculturation of Japanese Americans and their increasing acceptance of an individualistic as opposed to a collective view, there may be more overt dialogue and also disagreement among the children of Japanese American elders.

Disclosure and Consent

In Japan, when the diagnosis is that a disease is terminal and the prognosis is poor, the details of the truth may be kept from the patient. For most Japanese Americans, however, this approach, in general, would not be necessary because of their familiarity with Western ethics regarding truth telling. It is advisable early in the clinical relationship to explore each patient's preferences regarding disclosure of serious clinical findings and to reconfirm these wishes at intervals.

Gender Issues

In a very traditional Japanese American family, home matters are managed by the wife and "outside" work matters are managed by the husband. However, with the increasing acculturation of the Japanese American family and the gradually changing views of women in Japan, it becomes difficult to make generalizations.

End-of-Life Decision Making and Care Intensity

End-of-life care discussions should be approached with courteous respect. The competent older Japanese American woman may still wish to defer decision making to her husband or oldest son, depending on the family's traditional values. In an acculturated family where individual decisions are valued over those of the group, the competent elder would probably make the decisions for end-of-life care.

In the presence of a terminal illness, a *shikata ga nai* or "it cannot be helped" view may be held, making it sometimes easier for open discussions of death and dying. This view essentially removes the blame or feeling of failure from the person and the family. In general, because of the importance in Japanese thinking of dying intact and the difficulty in understanding "brain death," discussion of organ transplantation may be difficult to approach with a very traditional Japanese family.

> *The importance in Japanese culture of dying intact may make discussion of organ transplantation difficult.*

With respect to nursing home placement, Japanese Americans are less likely than their white counterparts to use nursing homes for their parents. However, they have a higher rate of nursing home use than do other Asian American groups.

Use of Advance Directives

The degree to which advance directives may be openly discussed depends on the degree of acculturation of the Japanese American elder. It is customarily said that the Japanese are born Shinto but die Buddhist. Shintoism may not favor open and active discussion on advance directives because thoughts about dying and death are considered negative and contaminating. Shintoism places emphasis on purity and cleanliness. The implication is that very early discussion of advance directives in an elder's life may not be effective. However, since it is commonly said that the Japanese die Buddhist, discussion of advance directives near the end of an elder's life may be effective. One study of advance directives in nursing home residents found that Japanese residents were more likely than other ethnic groups to request no-code status. Perhaps a *shikata ga nai* or "it cannot be helped" general view influenced the decision.

| CASE STUDY **1** | **Filial Piety** |

Objective
1. Discuss the impact and interplay of traditional values including filial piety, family honor, and avoidance of shame on decision making for elders in Japanese American families.

Mrs. Tanaka is an 85-year-old Japanese female who came to America from Japan in 1936 when she was 18 years old. She speaks very little English because, during her lifetime, she has associated mostly with the Japanese-speaking community. Widowed for 10 years, she lives alone in her home, but is now reaching the point where she is unable to live independently. Her medical history is significant for end-stage Parkinson's disease and osteoarthritis of both knees. She used a walker until her recent hip fracture from a fall at home 2 months ago. Through a trial of inpatient and outpatient rehabilitation, she has advanced, at most, to ambulating with a walker with moderate supervision. As a consequence, she has some functional urinary incontinence and has had some very rare stool incontinence. Although she does not have dementia, she has dysphagia. She requires a minced food consistency with liquids thickened to honey consistency.

Mrs. Tanaka has three children. The oldest son is the chief executive officer of a communications company that was recently involved in a hostile takeover of another company. His wife is an attorney. The second oldest is a daughter, a Japanese high school teacher who did postgraduate work in Japan for 3 years, and during her sojourn in Japan, married a Japanese national who now teaches Japanese at a community college. Mrs. Tanaka's daughter and son-in-law live an hour's drive from her home. The youngest son is an elite hairdresser who is contemplating opening his own business. He is not married and lives in a rented studio near his mother.

Dr. Cadigan is a Caucasian internist 2 years into his group practice. He is enthusiastic and idealistic. He has immensely enjoyed his practice thus far and, by chance, has been spared working with any difficult patients or families. On his schedule, he notices that Mrs. Tanaka will be coming with her oldest son.

The reason Mrs. Tanaka and her oldest son visit the clinic is to fill out an application form for nursing home placement. Dr. Cadigan says to both the son and Mrs. Tanaka, "So you are interested in a nursing home?" The son replies, "Yes," but Mrs. Tanaka is quiet. Dr. Cadigan senses a mixture of sadness and resignation on her part. When they are alone,

Dr. Cadigan discusses nursing home placement with Mrs. Tanaka, and she says it is the best decision for the whole family and that she would like to go into a nursing home. After a physical examination is performed, Dr. Cadigan tells the son that the form will be ready by the end of the week.

The following day as Dr. Cadigan is getting ready to see his first patient, the nurse interrupts him with a call from Mrs. Tanaka's daughter. The daughter relates that Mrs. Tanaka really does not want to go to the nursing home and should not go against her will. She further states that Mrs. Tanaka finds it difficult to assert her wishes and that this is consistent with her upbringing. Mrs. Tanaka's daughter feels it is important for the physician to understand the situation in a cultural context and wants to further discuss the situation on the phone. As Dr. Cadigan is about to discuss the issue, he recalls that the Health Insurance Portability and Accountability Act (HIPAA) privacy rule does not allow him to freely discuss his office encounter with Mrs. Tanaka's daughter, and he kindly ends the call.

Near the end of Dr. Cadigan's busy week, Mrs. Tanaka visits the clinic with her daughter. Mrs. Tanaka is quiet. Dr. Cadigan asks her privately if she wants to go to a nursing home. She answers, "Whatever is best, doctor, I do." Dr. Cadigan presses on and asks her what is deep down in her thoughts. Mrs. Tanaka relates that, "If not needed, I prefer to stay home, but if cannot help, I will go." Realizing that more time will be needed to assist the Tanakas in their decision making, Dr. Cadigan asks for a family conference to be arranged to discuss various options.

A meeting is set up. Mrs. Tanaka, her two sons and daughter, as well as her daughter-in-law and son-in-law arrive. Dr. Cadigan asks if having Mrs. Tanaka remain in her home is an arrangement the family will consider, because she will need some type of arranged assistance. Her daughter and son-in-law suggest that she live with the oldest son in his home. The oldest son states that this arrangement is not an option and that their mother is better off in a nursing home. His tone of voice becomes argumentative. The daughter and youngest son remind him that filial piety is important and ask him to look into his heart to see what their mother has done for them. They remind the oldest son that it is his obligation and he should honor the family name, especially because as the oldest son, he has inherited the family home. The oldest son curtly states that the youngest son has already damaged the family name. The oldest son is asked by his sister to stop discussing topics irrelevant to the situation. In the meantime, Mrs. Tanaka has remained quiet and gazes down. When asked her opinion, she answers, "Whatever is best, I'll do." Dr. Cadigan feels that nothing will be solved today. He thinks the best thing to do is to discuss options and request another family meeting after the family has had time for more thought and discussion.

Questions:

1. What are some cultural issues that come into play in this family meeting?
2. What is the impact of filial piety on various family members in this scenario?
3. What traditional values, for example filial piety, honoring the family name, and not bringing shame to the family, do the oldest son and daughter share? Which do they not seem to share?
4. What is Mrs. Tanaka's approach to family conflict? How might this reflect her cultural values as an older Japanese American?
5. The family home has been transferred to the oldest son, in keeping with Mrs. Tanaka's traditional values. What are Mrs. Tanaka's expectations with regard to how she will be cared for in later years?

Dr. Cadigan discusses options with the family such as having Mrs. Tanaka attend a day program with her evenings supervised by the family who might rotate the evening supervisions or hire caregivers. Other considerations they discuss include having Mrs. Tanaka stay home with a professional caregiver. If she qualifies, PACE (Program of All-Inclusive Care for the Elderly) is a consideration, but she will still need supervision in the evenings. Other considerations might be for Mrs. Tanaka to live with her daughter and son-in-law in their home or with her youngest son. A nursing home, as originally requested by the oldest son, is still an option, of course. All of these options would require reviewing Mrs. Tanaka's financial situation.

After discussing the various options for Mrs. Tanaka, Dr. Cadigan asks the family and Mrs. Tanaka to explore them. At the next family meeting, Dr. Cadigan is happy when he is told that everyone has agreed on the following arrangement. Mrs. Tanaka will stay in her own home and attend a day program during the day. At night, her daughter, son, and son-in-law will rotate the evenings. The oldest son has decided not to participate in this arrangement, but he will contribute financially for hired help to cover his turns. The extra hired help allows his siblings to take breaks from caregiving.

The final consensus decision is a good one overall, because to a certain degree it meets everyone's cultural outlook and expectations. The oldest son, from whom much was expected, is contributing significantly, but in a financial way. Mrs. Tanaka's daughter, with a traditional view of filial piety, is contributing as well, as is Mrs. Tanaka's youngest son. Mrs. Tanaka, who wanted to avoid conflict and confrontation and would not directly express her wishes, is now able to remain in her home, as she desired.

| CASE STUDY **2** | **End of Life—Beginning of a Trip** |

Objectives
1. Review Japanese American traditional practices toward visiting elders and gift giving.
2. Discuss Japanese American Buddhist religious beliefs toward death and dying.

Mr. Suzuki is an 88-year-old *nissei,* a second-generation Japanese American. His wife is 80 years old and a first-generation Japanese American. With a medical history significant for hypertension, Mr. Suzuki was diagnosed with pancreatic cancer 1 month ago. He has lost 35 pounds in the last 2 months, and his functional status has declined to the point where he needs moderate assistance with ambulation, dressing, grooming, and bathing. Although he is able to feed himself, he becomes weary and then needs to be fed by others. Dr. Brook, his physician, has recommended home hospice. At first reluctant with the unfamiliar, both Mr. Suzuki and his wife are finally receptive to home hospice after a month of encouragement from their daughter, who is an intensive care nurse.

The hospice nurse arranges a home visit for an initial evaluation prior to entering into hospice. She arrives at their doorstep at the scheduled time, and Mrs. Suzuki opens the door and invites her in. Mrs. Suzuki seems surprised when the nurse comes right in, but the hospice nurse attributes this to her newly dyed reddish brown hair that has a shimmer to it. The home is clean with white carpeting. Mr. Suzuki's sister is visiting from Japan and bows her head respectfully to the nurse as she enters the home. Mr. Suzuki is lying on the living room sofa. He is thin, weak, and appears closer to death than the hospice nurse had anticipated over the phone. He takes narcotics on a scheduled basis and is remarkably pain free. He has been eating primarily soft rice, and lately his wife has been mixing it with fermented soy beans, or *natto,* for extra nutrition. With a barely audible voice, he thanks the nurse for coming and seems genuinely grateful. The nurse performs a hospice intake evaluation. At the end of the evaluation, Mrs. Suzuki gives the nurse a small gift box explaining that it is a gift from Japan brought by Mr. Suzuki's sister. Because the gift is perishable, Mrs. Suzuki recommends consuming it in a day or two. Thrilled with the gift, the nurse tears off the meticulously wrapped paper and opens the box. In it are five beautiful teacakes in the form of flowers, fruits, and leaves. She joyously thanks the Suzukis and gently places one cake in her mouth. As soon as her teeth sink into the cake, however, the nurse realizes that the texture is not quite to her liking and the cake seems a bit too sweet. After taking one bite, she graciously places the rest of the cake back in the box and thanks them again. As she concludes her visit, she says that she will be calling to set up another visit. Mrs. Suzuki sees her to the door and waits at the doorstep until the nurse is actually in the car and ready to drive away. Mrs. Suzuki bows down again.

A few days later, after a care plan has been written, the hospice nurse calls to make arrangements for a follow-up home visit. Mrs. Suzuki seems a little hesitant and says that her husband is doing well. The hospice nurse offers to call again in a few days. The following day, the hospice nurse receives a call from Mr. Suzuki's daughter who says that Mr. Suzuki stopped eating 2 days ago, but seems comfortable. Should he require something for pain, however, she would appreciate it if Dr. Brook could order something because Mr. Suzuki can no longer take oral medications. Casually mentioning that Mrs. Suzuki had declined a visit, the hospice nurse says that she will contact Dr. Brook. The daughter responds that she has talked with her mother, and that they are all receptive to another home visit.

Question:

1. What are some cultural insights that may help on home visits to a relatively traditional Japanese family?

The home care nurse arranges a visit to the Suzuki home. When she arrives, she removes her shoes and enters the home. Mr. Suzuki's breathing is shallow, and his blood pressure is barely palpable. The hospice nurse feels he will pass on soon. Away from the patient, she tells this to his wife. Mrs. Suzuki calls their daughter to come home and also requests their Buddhist priest's presence. The hospice nurse assures the family that Mr. Suzuki seems comfortable. As the hospice nurse begins to put away her stethoscope, she sees that Mrs. Suzuki, who is near her husband, is weeping. The nurse notices that Mr. Suzuki is no longer breathing. When she checks his pulse, she finds he is pulseless and without heart tones on auscultation. Mr. Suzuki has quietly and peacefully passed on. When the Suzuki's daughter subsequently arrives, the hospice nurse gives her condolences, and the daughter thanks her graciously. The daughter says that she can take care of things now and proceeds to tell her mother that their priest should be coming soon. She mentions that she hopes Mr. Suzuki's trip will be easy. The nurse knows that the community mortuary is only a block away, is puzzled by the "trip," and hopes that it is an easy one.

Question:

1. What are some of the insights that might help in working with Japanese Americans with Buddhist beliefs?

The hospice nurse leaves. She feels fulfilled because Mr. Suzuki has had a good and peaceful death. She also has become interested in Japanese culture and is thinking about a trip to Japan next spring to view cherry blossoms.

Marianne K. G. Tanabe, MD

References

Bisignani, JD. *Japan Handbook*. 2nd ed. Chico, CA: Moon Publications, Inc; 1993.

Braun, KL, Browne CV. Perceptions of dementia, caregiving, and help seeking among Asian and Pacific Islander Americans. *Health Soc Work* 1998; 23(4):262–274.

Braun KL, Nichols R. Death and dying in four Asian American cultures: a descriptive study. *Death Stud* 1997;21(4):327–359.

Campbell R, Brody EM. Women's changing roles and help to the elderly: attitudes of women in the United States and Japan. *Gerontologist* 1985;25(6): 584–592.

Curb JD, Reed DM, Miller FD, et al. Health status and life style in elderly Japanese men with a long life expectancy. *J Gerontol* 1990;45(5):S206-S211.

Donahue RP, Abbott RD, Reed DM, et al. Alcohol and hemorrhagic stroke: The Honolulu Heart Program. *JAMA* 1986;255(17):2311–2314.

Edward B, Philip R. *World Civilization*. 5th ed, vol. 2. New York: W.W. Norton and Company, Inc; 1974.

Goldstein BZ, Tamura K. *Japan and America: A Comparative Study in Language and Culture*. Rutland, VT: Charles E. Tuttle Company; 1975.

Kinoshita J, Palevsky N. *Gateway to Japan*. 2nd ed. Tokyo, Japan: Kodansha International Ltd; 1992.

Koyano, Wataru. Japanese attitudes toward the elderly: a review of research findings. *J Cross-Cultural Gerontol* 1989;4:335–345.

Launer J, Masaki K, Petrovitch H, et al. The association between midlife blood pressure levels and late-life cognitive function: The Honolulu-Asia Aging Study. *JAMA* 1995;274(23):1846–1851.

Lebra TS. *Japanese Patterns of Behavior*. Honolulu, HI: University Press of Hawaii; 1976.

McBride M, Morioka-Douglas N, Yeo G, eds. *Aging and Health: Asian and Pacific Islander American Elders*. 2nd ed. Stanford GEC Working Paper #3. Stanford, CA: Stanford Geriatric Education Center; 1996.

McDermott JF Jr, Tseng W, Maretzki TW, et al. *People and Cultures of Hawaii: A Psychocultural Profile*. Honolulu, HI: School of Medicine and University of Hawaii Press; 1980.

McLaughlin LA, Braun KL. Asian and Pacific Islander cultural values: considerations for health care decision making. *Health Soc Work* 1998; 23(2):116–126.

Palafox N, Warren A, eds. *Cross-Cultural Caring, A Handbook for Health Care Professionals in Hawaii.* Honolulu, HI: Transcultural Health Care Forum; John A. Burns School of Medicine, University of Hawaii; 1980.

Rantanen T, Guralnik JM, Foley D, et al. Midlife hand grip strength as a predictor of old age disability. *JAMA* 1999;281(6):558–560.

Ross GW, Abbott RD, Petrovitch H, et al. Frequency and characteristics of silent dementia among elderly Japanese-American men: The Honolulu-Asia Aging Study. *JAMA* 1997;277(10):800–805.

Tomita, S. The consideration of cultural factors in the research of elder mistreatment with an in-depth look at the Japanese. *J Cross-Cultural Gerontol* 1994; 9:39–52.

Vaughn G, Kiyasu E, McCormick WC. Advance directive preferences among subpopulations of Asian nursing home residents in the Pacific Northwest. *J Am Geriatr Soc.* 2000;48(5):554–557.

White L, Petrovitch H, Ross GW, et al. Prevalence of dementia in older Japanese-American men in Hawaii: The Honolulu-Asia Aging Study. *JAMA* 1996; 276(12): 955–960.

CHAPTER 8

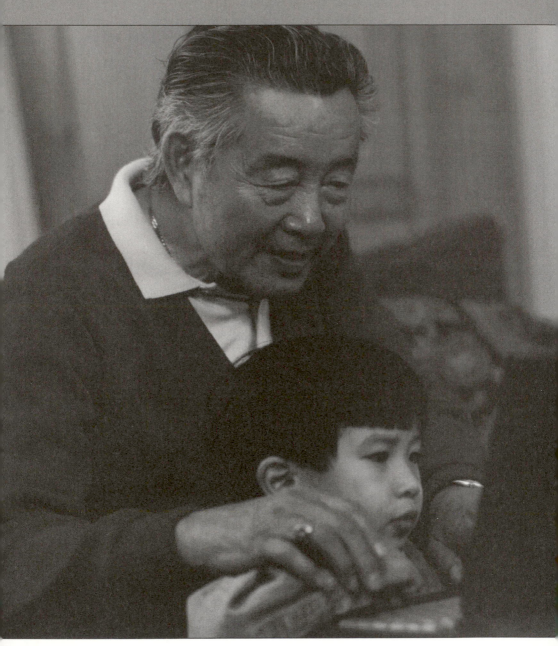

Older Chinese Americans

Doorway Thoughts

The key concepts discussed in this text are "doorway thoughts"—factors that the culturally sensitive and competent practitioner reflects upon before walking through the doorway of any examining, consultation, or hospital room. Practitioners who obtain a basic understanding of the background and beliefs of the patients they care for will likely establish more therapeutic relationships and avoid cultural missteps.

The Chinese population in the United States is diverse, with intra group variations in dialects, education level, immigration period, and degrees of acculturation. While the spoken language can sound very different across dialects, the written language is by and large uniform, and serves as a way of communicating among Chinese people from different regions.

While the general concepts about Chinese elders that are described here provide useful background information, clinicians must personalize care to the individual patient. Clinicians must ensure that generalizations not become stereotypes that are used in defining individual patients. When in doubt, it is always advisable to ask open-ended questions to explore the patient's understanding and paradigm about his/her condition.

Preferred Cultural Terms

The preferred term for the patients' cultural and ethnic identity is *Chinese* or *Chinese American*. To be more general, use the term *Asian*, but not *Oriental,* which can have a negative connotation. It is always helpful to be more specific and inquire what the patient's dialect is, e.g., Cantonese, Mandarin, Toishan, Taiwanese, or Shanghainese.

Formality of Address

Chinese patients tend to prefer a more formal and hierarchical approach to address. The younger person respects the elder and has respect for authority, including that of the physician. In general, the clinician should address the Chinese patient by using his or her formal title (e.g., Mr., Mrs.) and surname. As a relationship with the patient becomes established, it becomes appropriate to ask the patient if he or she wishes to be addressed in any other way. Chinese patients will address the physician as "Doctor" or "Dr. Smith."

Language and Literacy

Because of immigration patterns and policies, older Chinese immigrants are likely to have been unskilled laborers, whereas newer immigrants and those of younger generations are mostly skilled professionals. The husband may speak English well because of work requirements, whereas the wife may speak little English if she is a homemaker. However, clinicians may also encounter a small group of older Chinese immigrants who are well educated and fluent in English, who established their careers in the United States and subsequently brought their families over from China. In this case, the older person may know more English and be more acculturated than the younger family members.

Respectful Nonverbal Communication

Chinese patients tend to be polite and may smile and nod; however, nodding does not necessarily indicate agreement or even understanding of medical facts. It is important to check with the patient or the family and ask, "We reviewed quite a bit of material; do you have any questions? Can you repeat in your own words what we have just talked about?"

History of Immigration

The Chinese have a long history in the United States. From 1850 to 1860, sojourner males (ratio of immigrant men to women 27:1) migrated from southern China to "Gold Mountain" (the literal translation of the Chinese characters for today's San Francisco). They sustained brutal living and working conditions, violence, and discriminatory legislation in the 1870s. In 1882 the Chinese Exclusion Act banned the immigration of Chinese laborers, which resulted in declining immigration through the 1920s. Between 1920 and 1940 immigration restrictions eased slightly, although the 1924

Immigration Act excluded all Asians. During this period, families merged in urban Chinatowns. In 1943, all 15 Chinese Exclusion Acts were repealed, and a law was passed allowing "alien" wives to immigrate. More than 9,000 Chinese wives immigrated to the United States, ushering in an era of increased educational attainment and high birthrates, although employment discrimination continued. In the 1950s a new immigration act was passed, favoring persons with kin in the United States. By 1960 the ratio of Chinese men to women in the United States equalized. The 1970s and 1980s saw the development of two distinct Chinese American communities: one suburban and well educated, the other more urban, with little education and low income. At the same time, immigration of Chinese from Vietnam also increased. There was heavy immigration from mainland China, Hong Kong, and Taiwan. Many older Chinese adults also immigrated as followers of children. In the 1990s, there was a resurgence of anti-immigration bias but also increasing diversity within the Chinese American community.

The history of Chinese immigration into the United States has resulted in wide economic and educational diversity within the Chinese American community.

Degree of Acculturation

There is a broad spectrum of acculturation among Chinese Americans, ranging from very traditional among first-generation immigrants to the complete acculturation of those whose families have been in North America for several generations. The best approach is to ask each patient individually about his or experience. Initial questions could include "Where were you born?" and "How long have you lived in this country?" If the clinician is unsure how acculturated the patient is, it is all right to admit ignorance by saying, "I have had limited experience taking care of Chinese patients. I have noticed that some Chinese patients are very traditional, whereas others are more westernized. Which group do you believe you belong to?" It is a good idea to ask the patient for specific examples that support his or her reply.

Extended family structures wherein two or three generations live in the same household are more common among recent immigrants than among acculturated families. In Chinese tradition, the wife is expected to become part of husband's family.

Tradition and Health Beliefs

Chinese patients may prefer being cared for by Chinese physicians, simply because of the cultural connection and common language. Chinese physicians may also be more knowledgeable about the Chinese elder's paradigm of health and illness, as well as his or her use of complementary medical modalities, such as acupuncture or herbal medicine. However, Chinese American elders are also accustomed to working with non-Chinese clinicians.

The use of home and folk remedies is very common. Such treatments are generally used first, especially for chronic conditions and minor ailments. The use of Western treatments in conjunction with traditional approaches is also common and may be reserved for more acute conditions or used later during the course of an illness. Some Chinese elders may return to their country of origin to receive such "mixed" treatments. It is less common for Chinese elders to use either traditional or Western treatments exclusively.

In general, traditional Chinese people believe that most illnesses are caused by an imbalance of *qi* (vital force or energy) and *yin* and *yang* in the body. Mental illness is thought to be due to lack of harmony of emotions or, in some cases, to be caused by evil spirits. Mental wellness occurs when psychological and physiologic functions are integrated. Genetic defects are usually blamed on the mother, generally something she did or ate. Health is maintained by balancing *yin-yang* not only in the body but also in the environment. According to Chinese tradition, it is important to maintain harmony with body, mind, and spirit, as well as with family and friends.

The sick role is a common behavior among Chinese patients. Family members are expected to care for the patient, and the patient may take a passive role in his or her illness.

Some Chinese fear having blood drawn, believing that it will weaken the body; many are averse to donating blood. Many will avoid surgery, believing that the body needs to stay intact so that the soul will have a place to live during future visits to earth. This stems from a belief in reincarnation, that is, that the soul may return to earth either in the same or a different physical shape.

Chinese patients may not be accustomed to eating Western food. When managing Chinese patients in a hospital or in a nursing home, it may be helpful to allow family members to bring food from home. Depending on the illness, family members may bring in foods that have "cold" or "hot" qualities to help remedy the illness. Foods are thought to have medicinal purposes, and food parts correspond to healing of body parts; for example, it is thought that eating fish eyes will improve vision. Food plays an important role in mediating health. Fluids (hot tea, soups, and soupy rice or *congee*) are consumed in abundance, especially when a person is ill.

Culture-Specific Health Risks

There is little specific information regarding the health status of Chinese Americans. However, the degree to which immigrants have adopted the culture and behaviors of Western society may have impacted their health in many cases. For example, comparison of illness patterns among Chinese Americans and among Chinese who live in mainland China, Hong King, or Singapore shows an increased rate of cancer of the breast, colon, and prostate in the Chinese Americans.

In China and Japan, stroke has been a principal cause of mortality for the past few decades. Ischemic stroke is more prevalent than hemorrhagic stroke in the Chinese population. By comparison, studies indicate that Chinese individuals living in North America have a lower risk of coronary artery disease than do individuals of South Asian and European descent.

There is a higher prevalence of hepatitis B among Chinese Americans born in Asia, where in many places hepatitis is endemic.

There is a higher prevalence of hepatitis B among Chinese Americans born in Asia, where in many places hepatitis is endemic. The incidence of active tuberculosis is also higher for Asians and Pacific Islanders born outside of the United States. In 1990, this incidence was 10 times that of the general U.S. population.

Chinese Americans have the highest rates of nasopharyngeal cancer (a type of head and neck cancer) in the United States. Men of Asian origin (e.g., Chinese, Korean, Filipino, and Japanese) also have the highest age-adjusted incidence rates of liver cancer in the United States. These rates are much higher than the overall rates in the United States but are lower than the incidence rates in their countries of origin. Among Chinese individuals in the United States who were born in Asia, 80% of liver cancer is associated with chronic hepatitis B infection.

Depression among Chinese American elders is underdiagnosed and undertreated. Chinese American women aged 65 years and older have three times the suicide rate of white women in the United States. Among women older than 75, the rate is seven times that of white women. The majority of Chinese American suicide victims are foreign born. Chinese American elders tend not to communicate the intent to commit suicide.

Vascular dementia is prevalent among Chinese American elders, possibly more prevalent than Alzheimer's disease in this group. This could be due to a relatively higher rate of hypertension. Thalassemia and glucose-6-dehydrogenase deficiency is also higher among Chinese Americans.

Approaches to Decision Making

In general, Chinese culture emphasizes and values family involvement and group decision making, rather than individual autonomy. However, with different degrees of acculturation, this varies among individual patients. The Chinese American population is a patriarchal society; the oldest males tend to make decisions, especially for young females. For older people, the eldest son may assume decision-making responsibility. But because women tend to be the caregivers, the family commonly makes decisions as a group.

Disclosure and Consent

Chinese culture emphasizes the implicit rather than the explicit, so that some concepts are presumed to be understood rather than stated. If the patient does not want to clarify certain statements, seek help from a family member.

Because the patient is already suffering from the illness, it is considered unnecessary, rude, and inappropriate to burden him or her further by discussing the nature of the disease. The patient does not require full knowledge because the family will make the necessary decisions.

Cancer appears to be an unspeakable diagnosis from which Chinese patients are usually shielded.

Studies indicate that although Chinese and U.S. internists are almost equally likely to disclose a diagnosis of terminal AIDS, Chinese internists are far less likely than their U.S. counterparts to disclose a diagnosis of cancer.

Cancer appears to be an unspeakable diagnosis from which Chinese patients are usually shielded. It is always helpful to ask the patient, "If there should be a serious diagnosis or condition, would you like me to tell you directly? Or would you rather I speak to your family?" The clinician should try to identify a family member who is trusted by the patient to make decisions and to serve as the health care proxy or agent.

Gender Issues

Chinese society tends to be patriarchal. Depending on the degree of acculturation, older Chinese males may relate better with male physicians. It is important to take cues from the patient.

In the traditional Chinese community, gay and lesbian relationships may not be acknowledged.

End-of-Life Decision Making and Care Intensity

Concepts of appropriate palliative care may vary among Chinese Americans. For example, in Hong Kong most critically ill patients are sent to the hospital, even if death is anticipated and no active resuscitation or life support is intended. In one Taiwanese study, advanced age, having children, and being unable to take anything by mouth were found to be predictive of cancer patients' returning home to die.

There may be a certain degree of superstition when it comes to discussing death and dying. For example, the Chinese word for the number "four" sounds similar to the word "death," therefore four is considered an unlucky number. Also, the very act of speaking about death may be unlucky and considered by some to invite death. As a result, some Chinese patients may use proverbs or symbolic language to discuss death rather than the actual word.

Use of Advance Directives

Data related to attitudes about advance directives among Chinese Americans are scarce. However, data from studies of various other Chinese communities in China, Taiwan, and Hong Kong indicate that attitudes about do-not-resuscitate (DNR) orders vary among regions (e.g., Taiwan versus Hong Kong). In general, DNR orders are usually in the form of verbal consents rather than written agreements. There may be an element of avoiding written consent in order to avoid blame or bad luck. Some Chinese patients may choose to ask the physician to make the decisions on their behalf; for example, some may say, "Doctor, you know what is best." The attitude toward death and dying among Chinese patients may vary widely, and it is important to assess and communicate with each patient individually.

CASE STUDY **1**	**Listen to Me; I Am the Patient**

Objectives

1. Discuss the importance of ascertaining the level of acculturation for each individual patient, as well as caregivers.
2. Describe the impact of the concept of filial piety on the actions of the daughters in this scenario.

Dr. Caroline Huang, a general internist in a teaching hospital, is a first-generation Chinese American who speaks Mandarin and English fluently. She is 3 years into practice and has an established panel of primary care patients. She works on a general medical ward, teaches students and residents, and works closely with an interdisciplinary team of nurses, nurse practitioners, social workers, and physical therapists.

Dr. Yang is a 90-year-old Chinese American male retired physician who came to the United States in his twenties. He received an American medical education and knows many of the senior physicians in the hospital. He married his wife through an arranged marriage and they have four devoted daughters. All of his children grew up in China and immigrated to the United States much later than Dr. Yang. Culturally, therefore, they are less Americanized and more traditionally Chinese. Dr. Yang has coronary artery disease, hypertension, osteoporosis, chronic obstructive pulmonary disease, acute chronic renal failure, and mild hearing impairment. Because of his renal failure and his refusal to undergo dialysis, he has become progressively more frail and has fallen and broken his hip. His four daughters take turns to be at his bedside, cater to his needs, and anxiously ask questions of Dr. Huang. They want to know whether Dr. Yang will need hip surgery and whether he can tolerate it. The daughters also state that Dr. Huang must do everything she can to restore Dr. Yang's health.

During the hospitalization, Dr. Huang spends considerable time and energy answering the daughters' questions outside the patient's room, because the daughters are very anxious about their father's condition. Dr. Yang often appears sleepy and answers questions slowly. When Dr. Huang goes to her patient's bedside, Dr. Yang angrily exclaims, "Don't listen to them! They don't know anything. You must talk to me. I am the patient."

Questions:

1. In this scenario, issues of acculturation play a prominent role. What are some of the unusual issues of acculturation brought out in this scenario and what impact do they have on Dr. Yang's care?

2. When the daughters tell Dr. Huang, "You must do everything," what traditional aspects of Chinese culture are being expressed?

Dr. Yang explains to his doctor that even though he is weak and hearing impaired, he knows about his condition and his high risk for surgical repair. He also demands that his medical background and knowledge be respected over the lay opinions of his daughters. He states that he does not want to be resuscitated if he should suffer a cardiopulmonary arrest, and quotes literature about advanced age and renal failure being poor prognostic factors. After 2 days, he suddenly becomes more short of breath and tachypneic and is diagnosed of a presumed pulmonary embolism.

The family surrounds the patient and asks Dr. Huang, "Isn't there anything you can do to save him?" Dr. Huang explains that Dr. Yang is a physician, knows his own body and mind, and has expressed wishes for no surgical interventions and no resuscitation, given his progressive medical illnesses. Dr. Huang emphasizes that the patient's autonomy must be respected and that the family should not feel guilty about Dr. Yang's dying.

The daughters express a Chinese proverb, loosely translated as "As long as there is the wooded mountain, fear not that there will be no logs to burn." They explain this means that every effort should be made to revive the patient in the hopes that he gets better. Dr. Huang counters with a different Chinese proverb, "It is better to be broken jade than untouched clay." She explains that Dr. Yang would wish to preserve his wholeness and dignity rather than suffer at the end of his life. The daughters understand and request that Dr. Yang's pain continue to be treated and that he is kept comfortable in his last days.

| CASE STUDY **2** | **The Grateful Patient with Lotus Cakes** |

Objectives

1. Devise two culturally sensitive responses to a patient who intends to use alternative Eastern therapies.
2. Discuss Chinese Americans' traditional attitudes toward physicians and how this might affect provider-patient communication.

Dr. Judy Frame is a family physician in a large metropolitan center. She has been the primary care physician for the last 8 years for Mrs. Chan, a 70-year-old Chinese American woman. Mrs. Chan came from Hong Kong to the United States 35 years ago with her husband, a successful importer, and three children. She is a homemaker and speaks little English. Two months ago, Mrs. Chan came in for knee pain. Dr. Frame diagnosed osteoarthritis, and prescribed regular acetaminophen because Mrs. Chan has a history of peptic ulcer disease. Mrs. Chan is coming in today to follow-up with Dr. Frame.

She arrives with her youngest son, who does some translation during the interview. Dr. Frame asks how she is doing, and Mrs. Chan complains that she is having some stomach discomfort. Her symptoms started about 6 weeks ago. She is concerned that her sister came from Singapore and gave her a large box of food which, she worries, caused her present symptoms. She is particularly concerned that the dried mangoes caused her to have "high heat," or *huo-chi*, and are creating problems.

Question:

1. How would you respond in a culturally sensitive way to Mrs. Chan's concerns that her "chi" is not in balance?

Dr. Frame admits to Mrs. Chan that she does not know much about the Eastern system of chi, but that she understands disease from a Western framework, which she hopes is complementary. After reviewing the food contents in detail, Dr. Frame is able to convince her that the food was unlikely to have caused her present symptoms. Dr. Frame has to finish the interview because they are running out of time. She sends Mrs. Chan for blood tests and asks her to come back in a week. Mrs. Chan looks very grateful, smiles, and asks her son to thank Dr. Frame. She presents the doctor with some homemade peanut candies for Dr. Frame and her staff.

Next week Mrs. Chan returns. Her blood work is normal. Dr. Frame is somewhat perplexed and concerned that Mrs. Chan has a serious gastrointestinal pathology. She decides to begin again and retakes Mrs. Chan's history. When they review her medications, Mrs. Chan recounts that she is taking the medications Dr. Frame prescribed for her high blood pressure. On further questioning, she states she is not taking the acetaminophen because she tried one pill a couple of times and there was no effect. Dr. Frame asks what she did for her knee pain, and Mrs. Chan states that she is taking a "Chinese herbal medication" that she purchased at a Chinese grocery store. Luckily, her son brought the insert for the pills. A list of contents is written in English in one corner of the insert. Dr. Frame realizes that one of the ingredients is in fact a "cortisone" and is quite likely causing her dyspepsia.

Questions:
1. How would you approach Mrs. Chan's discontinuance of her acetaminophen and her use of an alternative herbal medication?
2. Why do you think that Mrs. Chan did not mention, without being asked, that Dr. Frame's treatment was ineffective?

Dr. Frame explains that the "herbal" medication Mrs. Chan is taking actually contains a strong pharmaceutical with possible side effects. The doctor acknowledges that alternative therapies can be quite useful, but she needs to know what Mrs. Chan is taking. The patient is quite happy to keep her informed and will discontinue the herbal medication. Dr. Frame explains that regular higher dose acetaminophen has a beneficial effect and that this is more "powerful" than using one small dose. Mrs. Chan is able to repeat this back to Dr. Frame. Mrs. Chan wonders about using acupuncture, and Dr. Frame happily agrees that this might be very helpful and will refer her to their physiotherapist who is Chinese American and is qualified to administer acupuncture. She contracts with Mrs. Chan that she will return in 2 weeks to discuss the effects of the combined acetaminophen and acupuncture treatments. Mrs. Chan is again effusively grateful and brings out lotus pastries for the doctor.

Cynthia X. Pan, MD
Janet Kushner Kow, MEd, MD, FRCPC

References
Chen MS. Health status of Chinese Americans: challenges and opportunities. Paper presented at: 7th International Conference of Health Problems Related to the Chinese; July 1–3, 1994.

Chin P. Chinese Americans. In: Lipson JG, Dibble SL, Minarik PA, eds. *Culture and Nursing Care: A Pocket Guide*. San Francisco, CA: UCSF Nursing Press; 1996;74–81.

Douglas KC, Fujimoto D. Asian Pacific elders: implications for health care providers. *Clin Geriatr Med* 1995;11(1):69–82.

Feldman MD, Zhang J, Cummings SR. Chinese and U.S. internists adhere to different ethical standards. *J Gen Intern Med* 1999;14(8):469–473

Gould-Martin K, Ngin C. Chinese Americans. In: Harwood A, ed. *Ethnicity and Medical Care*. Cambridge, MA: Harvard University Press; 1981:130–171.

Helman CG. *Culture, Health and Illness*. 3rd ed. Oxford, UK: Butterworth-Heinemann Ltd; 1994.

Hou L, Osei-Hyiaman D, Yu H, et al. Association of a 27-bp repeat polymorphism in ecNOC gene with ischemic stroke in Chinese patients. *Neurology* 2001;56(4): 490–496.

Huff RM, Kline MV. *Promoting Health in Multicultural Populations: A Handbook for Practitioners*. Thousand Oaks, CA: Sage Publishers; 1999.

Ip M, Gilligan T, Koenig B, et al. Ethical decision-making in critical care in Hong Kong. *Crit Care Med* 1998;26(3):447–451.

Lassiter S. *Multicultural Clients: A Professional Handbook for Health Care Providers and Social Workers*. Westport, CT: Greenwood; 1995:35–49.

Lin, TY. Psychiatry and Chinese culture. *Western J Med* 1983;139(6):862–867.

Liu JM, Lin WC, Chen YM, et al. The status of the do-not-resuscitate order in Chinese clinical trial patients in a cancer centre. *J Med Ethics* 1999;25(4): 309–314.

Lum OM. Health status of Asians and Pacific Islanders. *Clin Geriatr Med* 1995; 11(1):53–67.

Ma GX. Between two worlds: the use of traditional and Western health services by Chinese immigrants. *J Community Health* 1999;24(6):421–437.

Miyahara K, Kawamoto T, Sase K, et al. Cloning and structural characterization of the human endothelial nitric oxide synthase gene. *Eur J Biochem* 1994;223:719–726.

Rawl SM. Perspectives on nursing care of Chinese Americans. *J Holistic Nurs* 1992;10(1):6–17.

el-Serag HB. Epidemiology of hepatocellular carcinoma. *Clin Liver Dis* 2001;5(1):87–107.

Sue S, Zane N, Ito J. Alcohol drinking patterns among Asian and Caucasian Americans. *J Cross-Cultural Psychol* 1979;10:41-56.

Yee B, Weaver G. Ethnic minorities and health promotion: developing a culturally competent agenda. *Generations* 1994;18(1).

Yeo G. Ethical considerations in Asian and Pacific Island elders. *Clin Geriatr Med* 1995;11(1):139–151.

Yeo G, Gallagher-Thompson D. *Ethnicity and the Dementias*. Washington, DC: Taylor & Francis; 1996.

See also:

http:www.fcmsdocs.org/7healthstatus.html

http://www.goldsea.com/AAD/population

http://www.stanford.edu/group/ethnoger/

INDEX